S0-ANR-857

Maternal-Newborn Nursing

FIFTH EDITION

Clinical Handbook

Sally B. Olds, RNC, MS
Marcia L. London, RNC, MSN, NNP
Patricia W. Ladewig, PhD, RNC, NP

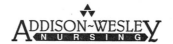

ADDISON-WESLEY NURSING

A Division of The Benjamin/Cummings Publishing Company, Inc.

Menlo Park, California • Reading, Massachusetts • New York
Don Mills, Ontario • Wokingham, U.K. • Amsterdam • Bonn • Paris
Milan • Madrid • Sydney • Singapore • Tokyo • Seoul • Taipei
Mexico City • San Juan, Puerto Rico

Executive Editor: *Patricia L. Cleary;* Managing Editor: *Wendy Earl;* Production Supervisor: *Sharon Montooth;* Editorial Assistant: *Marla Nowick;* Compositor and Page Designer: *Leigh Mclellan Design;* Art Coordinator: *David Novak;* Copy Editor: *Antonio Padial;* Proofreader: *Lorraine Newnam;* Indexer: *Sylvia Coates;* Senior Manufacturing Supervisor: *Merry Free Osborn;* Printer and Binder: *Banta Company;* Cover Printer: *New England Book Components;* Cover Quilt: *I See the Moon,* by Joy Baaklini

Copyright © 1996 by Addison-Wesley Nursing, A Division of The Benjamin/Cummings Publishing Company, Inc.

All rights reserved. No part of this publication may be reproduced, stored in a retrieval system, or transmitted, in any form or by any means, electronic, mechanical, photocopying, recording, or any other media or embodiments now known or hereafter to become known, without the prior written permission of the publisher. Manufactured in the United States of America. Published simultaneously in Canada.

Library of Congress Cataloging-in-Publication Data

Olds, Sally B., 1940–
    Maternal-newborn nursing clinical handbook / Sally B. Olds, Marcia L. London, Patricia W. Ladewig.
      p. cm.
    Includes bibliographical references and index.
    ISBN 0-8053-5614-2
    1. Maternity nursing—Handbooks, manuals, etc. I. London, Marcia L. II. Ladewig, Patricia W. III. Title.
    [DNLM: 1. Maternal-Child Nursing—handbooks. 2. Neonatal Nursing—handbooks. WY 49 044m 1995]
RG951.0433 1995
610.73'678—dc20
DNLM/DLC
for Library of Congress   95–44396
                                             CIP

1 2 3 4 5 6 7 8 9 10–BAM–99 98 97 96 95

Care has been taken to confirm the accuracy of information presented in this book. The authors, editors, and the publisher, however, cannot accept any responsibility for errors or omissions or for the consequences from application of the information in this book and make no warranty, express or implied, with respect to its contents.

The authors and publisher have exerted every effort to ensure that drug selections and dosages set forth in this text are in accord with current recommendation and practice at time of publication. However, in view of ongoing research, changes in government regulations, and the constant flow of information relating to drug therapy and drug reactions, the reader is urged to check the package inserts of all drugs for any change in indications of dosage and for added warnings and precautions. This is particularly important when the recommended agent is a new and/or infrequently employed drug.

Addison-Wesley Nursing
A Division of the Benjamin/Cummings Publishing Company, Inc.
2725 Sand Hill Road
Menlo Park, California 94025

Preface

Your assignment this morning when you enter the mother-baby unit as a nursing student (or a nurse new to the maternal-child area) is to provide care for four mothers and their babies. The first mother is a gravida 2, para 2, who had a cesarean birth early this morning under epidural anesthesia and also had an intrathecal narcotic to enhance her pain relief. Her baby will be coming from the admission nursery in an hour or so. The second mother is a primipara, 6 hours past birth, who is breastfeeding. The postpartum course is proceeding normally. The third mother is a 15-year-old primipara who is 10 hours past birth. She is breastfeeding and has yet to have a positive feeding experience. She is working hard to breastfeed, but her baby is very sleepy and somewhat uninterested in feeding. They are to be discharged in 2 hours, and the mother has no support available to her. The fourth mother is a gravida 4, para 4, who has just been moved from the birthing area. Her fundus tends to become boggy, and the lochia rubra has been moderate to heavy with some clots. She has an IV with 20 units of oxytocin (Pitocin) to stimulate uterine contractions.

As you organize your thoughts for today, think about your priorities. What special assessments and interventions will each mother and baby need? How will you assist the breastfeeding mothers? How will you help connect the 15-year-old to a support base? In the midst of all of the aspects of care that are needed, how will you provide the self-care and teaching information that each new family needs?

The *Maternal-Newborn Nursing Clinical Handbook* has been created to help you in situations just like these. The handbook provides succinct, pertinent information regarding the antepartum, intrapartum, newborn, and postpartum client. Each content area includes key information regarding medical therapy as well as nursing care information organized according to the nursing process. Critical nursing assessments and interventions are identified, and specific suggestions are given regarding documentation of care. In many sections, a special "Alert" heading signals the reader to watch for specific signs and symptoms.

In addition to serving as a resource for normal and selected complications of childbearing, the handbook includes practical features to assist the nurse. Procedures specific to the maternal-child clinical area are included to help you provide nursing care. Commonly used medications are presented in the drug guides. A specially developed appendix with Spanish translations of some key phrases used in the maternal-child area will assist the nurse who does not speak Spanish.

Although the handbook gives condensed information about each subject area, critical aspects of nursing practice have been presented. It is our hope that this book will enhance maternal-newborn nursing practice and help nurses provide safe, competent care to all mothers and babies.

We would like to express our appreciation to the Addison-Wesley team for their encouragement, support, and assistance. Patti Cleary, our editor, provided a special spark that fired the creative process. Marla Newick, editorial assistant, took on endless lists of tasks, organized monumental stacks of papers, and still endured with humor. We would also like to extend a special thank you to other faculty colleagues and professional nurses. Elizabeth Medina, Ph.D., associate professor of Spanish at Regis University in Denver, Colorado, provided the Spanish translation for the appendix. Marguerite McMillan Jackson, RN, doctoral candidate, CIC, FAAN, administrative director of the Medical Center, Epidemiology Unit, University of California, San Diego, reviewed the appendix related to new CDC recommendations (1995) and OSHA Bloodborne Pathogens Standard (1991). These women offered their special expertise, and we are most appreciative.

Finally, we would like to express our heartfelt appreciation to our nursing students, who brighten each day. By being with them, we gained an understanding of their struggle to master an evergrowing body of knowledge. We have incorporated many of their requests and ideas into the information that appears in this handbook. As always, it is our goal to provide a tool that students and practicing nurses will find helpful.

SBO
MLL
PAL

BRIEF CONTENTS

CONTENTS

PROCEDURES

APPENDICES

INDEX   357

PHOTOGRAPHIC CREDITS

CHAPTER 5

Figures 5–1, 5–2, and 5–9: © Elizabeth Elkin. Figures 5–5 and 5–6: Reprinted by permission of V. Dubowitz, M.D., Hammersmith Hospital, London, England.

CHAPTER 6

Figure 6–1: © Suzanne Arms Wimberley.

CHAPTER 7

Figure 7–3: © Anne Dowie/Addison-Wesley Publishing.
Figure 7–4: © Kathleen Cameron.

CHAPTER 8

Figure 8–4: © Amy H. Snyder.

CHAPTER 11

Figure 11–1: © Elizabeth Elkin.

ILLUSTRATORS

Kristin N. Mount, Nea Hanscomb, Joanne Bales/Precision Graphics, and George Kupfer/Left Coast Group.

CHAPTER 1

The Antepartum Client

OVERVIEW

Pregnancy generally lasts about nine calendar months, ten lunar months, 40 weeks, or 280 days. The woman's due date (date on which baby is expected) is calculated from the first day of her last menstrual period (LMP). In reality, conception actually occurs about 14 days before the start of her next menstrual period. Thus the actual time she is pregnant is about two weeks less, or 266 days.

Typically, pregnancy is discussed in terms of trimesters, which each last three calendar months. During the first trimester, the woman usually learns she is pregnant and may seek prenatal care. The first trimester is the time of primary organ development for the fetus.

The second trimester is considered the most tranquil for the pregnant woman. Morning sickness passes, and quickening (feeling the baby move) occurs.

In the third trimester the woman becomes anxious for the pregnancy to end. She may feel awkward because of her increasing weight and the physical and psychologic changes she experiences.

During the antepartal period nursing interventions focus primarily on client teaching and ongoing monitoring of the woman so that any potential complications are detected promptly. Teaching typically focuses on nutrition, on interventions to deal with the common discomforts of pregnancy, and on self-care activities indicated throughout pregnancy.

NORMAL PHYSICAL CHANGES OF PREGNANCY

Uterus

- Dramatic increase in size and weight.
- **Braxton Hicks contractions** begin by the end of the first trimester. These are rhythmic contractions of the uterus that are painless initially but become noticeable, and sometimes uncomfortable, toward term (the end of pregnancy). They are then referred to as "false labor." Braxton Hicks contractions are palpable during bimanual exam by the fourth month and palpable abdominally by the 28th week.

Cervix

- Glandular tissue increases in number and becomes hyperactive.
- Mucous plug is formed in cervix, which acts as a barrier to prevent ascending infection.
- Increased blood flow to cervix leads to softening (Goodell's sign) and bluish coloration (Chadwick's sign) (visible on speculum examination).

Ovaries

- Ovum production ceases.
- Corpus luteum persists and secretes hormones until weeks 10–12.

Vagina

- Increased vascularity produces bluish color (Chadwick's sign).
- Epithelium hypertrophies.

Breasts

- Increased size and nodularity; some increased tenderness.
- Superficial veins prominent.
- Increased pigmentation of areola and nipple.

- Colostrum is usually produced by week 12. (Colostrum is the antibody-rich forerunner of mature breast milk.) Women who are not visibly secreting colostrum need reassurance that they are producing it even if it is not evident.

Respiratory System

- Some hyperventilation occurs as pregnancy progresses.
- Increased tidal volume, decreased airway resistance.
- Diaphragm elevated, substernal angle increased.
- Breathing changes from abdominal to thoracic.

Cardiovascular System

- Blood volume increases about 45%.
- Decreased systemic and pulmonary vascular resistance.
- By weeks 24–28, cardiac output increases 30% to 50% over prepregnant levels; remains elevated for duration of pregnancy.
- Increased pulse rate.
- BP decreases slightly by second trimester; near prepregnant levels at term.
- Pressure of enlarging uterus on vena cava can interfere with blood return to the heart and cause dizziness, pallor, clamminess, and lowered BP. This condition is called vena caval syndrome or supine hypotensive syndrome. Research suggests that the uterus may also exert pressure on aorta and its collateral circulation, making the term *aortocaval compression* more accurate (Blackburn & Loper 1992). It is corrected by having woman lie on her side or with a wedge under the right hip.
- RBC and hemoglobin levels increase as does plasma level. Because plasma volume increases more, a **physiologic anemia of pregnancy** results, evident in an apparent decrease in hematocrit (Hct). Hct levels of 32% to 44% are considered normal.
- Leukocyte production increases to levels of 10,000–11,000/mm^3. Levels may reach 25,000/mm^3 during labor.
- Increased fibrin, fibrinogen, factors VII, VIII, IX, X.

Gastrointestinal System

- Nausea common; vomiting occurs occasionally.
- Ptyalism (excessive salivation) is an occasional problem.
- Intestines and stomach are displaced by uterus.
- Relaxed cardiac sphincter leads to reflux of acidic secretions, resulting in heartburn.
- Delayed gastric emptying leads to constipation.
- Hemorrhoids may develop.

Urinary Tract

- Increased pressure on the bladder from the growing uterus during the first and third trimesters leads to urinary frequency.
- Glomerular filtration rate (GFR) and renal plasma flow (RPF) increased.
- Increased incidence of glycosuria, which may be normal or may indicate gestational diabetes mellitus (see Chapter 2).

Skin and Hair

- Increased pigmentation of areola, nipples, vulva, linea nigra.
- Facial chloasma, a butterfly-shaped area of pigmentation over the face, may develop. Usually fades after childbirth. Called the "mask of pregnancy."
- Striae or stretch marks may develop on the abdomen, also on breasts and thighs.
- Vascular spider nevi, small, bright red elevations of the skin radiating from central body, may develop.
- Rate of hair growth may decrease.

Musculoskeletal System

- Joints of pelvis relax somewhat.
- Waddling gait develops because of changed center of gravity and accentuated lumbosacral curve.
- Separation of rectus abdominis muscle may occur, called diastasis recti.

SIGNS OF PREGNANCY

1. **Subjective (presumptive) changes.** Symptoms experienced by woman; may be caused by conditions other than pregnancy. They include the following: amenorrhea, nausea and vomiting, excessive fatigue, urinary frequency, changes in the breasts, quickening (mother's perception of fetal movement).

2. **Objective (probable) changes.** Signs perceived by the examiner; may be caused by conditions other than pregnancy. They include the following: changes in the pelvic organs such as Goodell's sign, Chadwick's sign, and Hegar's sign (softening of the isthmus, the area between the cervix and the body of the uterus); enlargement of the abdomen; Braxton Hicks contractions; uterine souffle (soft blowing sound heard when auscultating the abdomen, caused by blood pulsating through the placenta); changes in pigmentation of the skin (chloasma, linea nigra); abdominal striae; fetal outline palpable during examination; positive pregnancy test.

3. **Diagnostic (positive) changes.** Signs that are completely objective and caused only by pregnancy. They include the following: detection of fetal heartbeat, fetal movements detected by a trained examiner, and verification of a gestational sac or fetal parts and heartbeat through ultrasonography.

PSYCHOLOGIC RESPONSES OF THE MOTHER TO PREGNANCY

Unless the following responses are extreme or exaggerated, they are considered normal. In most cases the nurse can reassure the woman of the normality of the response and explain that it is related to hormonal changes and to the body's efforts to prepare for childbirth and parenting.

1. **Ambivalence.** Initially, even if pregnancy is planned, the mother may have mixed feelings about it. She may have concerns about her career, her relationship with her partner, financial implications, and role change. She may make comments such as "I thought I wanted a baby but now that I'm pregnant, I'm not so sure."

2. **Acceptance of pregnancy.** As the woman begins to accept the reality of the pregnancy she shows a high degree of tolerance for the discomforts she may experience in the first trimester. In the second trimester she may begin wearing maternity clothes. At about 17 to 21 weeks she will begin to perceive movement. She may make comments such as, "Feeling the baby move makes it all seem real" or "It's finally sinking in that I'm going to be a mother."

3. **Introversion.** The expectant woman typically becomes more inwardly focused, less interested in outside activities. She is using this time to plan and adjust. Her partner may see this as excluding him. She may say, "I never used to like to be alone but now I like having time to myself just to think and plan."

4. **Mood swings.** Mood swings from joy to sadness are common and difficult for the woman and her family. The woman often feels a great need for love and affection, but her partner, confused by her emotional changes, may react by withdrawing. She may say, "I'm not usually so emotional but lately any little thing can set me off."

5. **Changes in body image.** Typically the woman tends to feel somewhat negative about her body as pregnancy progresses. Her increasing abdomen coupled with the waddling gait of pregnancy may cause a woman to feel ungainly and unattractive. She may say, "I can't even see my feet anymore" or "I feel big as a house."

PSYCHOLOGIC TASKS OF THE MOTHER

Rubin (1984) identified the following developmental tasks of the mother:

1. **Ensuring safe passage through pregnancy, labor, and birth.** To meet this task she seeks competent prenatal care, practices good health behaviors and self-care activities, reads about childbirth, and gathers information.

2. **Seeking acceptance of this child by others.** The expectant woman seeks to gain support for the coming child from her partner and family. She will

also work to help her other children accept the coming baby.

3. **Seeking of commitment and acceptance of self as mother to the infant (binding-in).** After she perceives fetal movement (quickening) the mother begins to form bonds of attachment to the child, and he/she becomes more real. The woman may talk about the child as a separate person: "The baby was so active today! I don't think he (or she) appreciated the pizza last night."

4. **Learning to give of one's self on behalf of one's child.** The woman begins to develop patterns of self-denial and delayed personal gratification to meet the needs of her child. She may, for example, give up smoking or alcohol and make plans to adjust her personal schedule to spend more time with her child.

ANTEPARTAL ASSESSMENT

Critical Terms

Gravida: any pregnancy, regardless of duration.

Primigravida: a woman who is pregnant for the first time.

Multigravida: a woman who is pregnant for her second or any subsequent pregnancy.

Para: birth after 20 weeks' gestation, regardless of whether infant is alive or dead.

Multipara: a woman who has had two or more births at more than 20 weeks' gestation.

Note: in clinical practice care givers often refer to a woman who is pregnant for the first time as a primip (short for primipara). In reality the correct term would actually be nulligravida, but it is seldom used. A woman becomes a primipara after she has had one birth of more than 20 weeks' gestation. Thus the term could be used on postpartum.

Preterm labor: labor that occurs after 20 weeks but before the completion of 37 weeks of gestation.

Stillbirth: a fetus born dead after 20 weeks' gestation.

Client History

1. **Current pregnancy.** A form of notation is used to quickly describe a woman's pregnancy history. For example, a woman pregnant for the first time would be gravida 1, para 0 (or G1 P0). A woman pregnant for the second time who has one living child born at term and had one miscarriage (also called spontaneous abortion) would be gravida 2 para 1 abortion 1 (G2 P1 Ab1).

   Some agencies use a more detailed approach: Gravida means the same as in the previous example; para refers to the number of infants but is further divided to identify the number of **t**erm, **p**reterm, **a**bortions, and **l**iving children (TPAL). The woman pregnant for the first time would be gravida 1 para 0000 (sometimes listed as 10000, 1 for gravida, 0000 for para). The second woman would be gravida 2 para 1011, i.e., one term infant, no preterm, one abortion, one living child (21011).

   Other critical information:
   - LMP: first day of last normal menstrual period (helps to date pregnancy)
   - Presence of any problems or complications such as bleeding
   - Any discomforts, concerns, questions

2. **History of past pregnancies.** Number of pregnancies, abortions (spontaneous or therapeutic), living children, complications. This information helps care givers avoid unintentionally hurtful comments and alerts them to potential problems. For example, a woman with a history of preterm labor is at increased risk for preterm labor.

3. **Gynecologic history.** Detailed gynecologic history is obtained. Critical information includes information on contraceptive history (For example, an intrauterine device [IUD] in place is usually removed because it could cause spontaneous abortion. Also, a woman who becomes pregnant while on birth control pills may have difficulty identifying LMP); history of sexually transmitted infections (history of herpes, for example, might influence route for childbirth); history of abnormal Pap smears.

4. **Current and past medical history.** Provides information about woman's general state of health and health habits, any medical/surgical conditions that might affect the pregnancy, such as diabetes, heart disease, sickle-cell anemia. Also notes use of alcohol, cigarettes, drugs, exposure to teratogens, allergies, current medications, blood type and Rh factor, record of immunizations, especially rubella.

5. **Religious/cultural/occupational history.** Gives information about any cultural influences and any workplace hazards.

Partner's History

Information is obtained about the partner's age; health; current and past medical history; use of substances including alcohol, cigarettes, social drugs, etc; blood type and Rh factor; occupation; and attitude about the pregnancy.

High-Risk Pregnancy

Certain factors in the woman's history place her at increased risk for complications during her current pregnancy. These include smoking, maternal age less than 20, previous preterm birth, and so forth. Preexisting medical conditions such as maternal diabetes automatically place the woman in a higher risk category. After the history is obtained, most agencies use a form to rate the number of risk factors and obtain a score. **Women who fall into a high-risk category are monitored more closely for potential complications.**

Initial Prenatal Physical Examination

Critical nursing actions The nurse is responsible for the following assessments at the initial prenatal examination:

- Vital signs, including temperature, pulse, respirations, and blood pressure (some agencies omit temperature)
- Height and weight

The nurse also obtains the following:

- Urinalysis (to detect proteinuria, glycosuria, hematuria, etc)
- Blood for CBC, including hematocrit (to detect anemia) and differential, VDRL, ABO and Rh typing, Rubella titer (to detect whether the woman is immune to German measles), sickle-cell screen for clients of African descent, other lab tests as ordered

The nurse then remains in the room to assist the examiner with the physical exam, including the pelvic exam.

Critical elements of the initial physical examination

1. **Skin.** Color noted (to detect anemia, cyanosis, jaundice); edema noted (may be normal or could indicate pregnancy-induced hypertension); changes normally associated with pregnancy noted, such as chloasma, linea nigra, spider nevi.

2. **Neck.** Thyroid assessed; may enlarge slightly during pregnancy; marked enlargement, nodules, etc, could indicate hyperthyroidism or goiter and are assessed further.

3. **Lungs.** Inspection, palpation, auscultation should be normal with no adventitious sounds.

4. **Breasts.** Inspection and palpation performed. Normal changes of pregnancy noted; orange-peel skin, palpable nodule suggest possible carcinoma; redness indicates mastitis.

5. **Heart.** Rate, rhythm, and heart sounds noted; should be normal. Short systolic murmur common due to increased blood volume.

6. **Abdomen.** Inspection and palpation performed. Liver and spleen not palpable. Shows changes of pregnancy including enlargement, striae.
   a. Fundus (upper portion of uterus) palpable as follows:
      - 10–12 weeks—slightly above symphysis
      - 16 weeks—halfway between symphysis and umbilicus
      - 20 weeks—at umbilicus

- 28 weeks—three fingerbreadths above umbilicus
- 36 weeks—just below ensiform cartilage

b. Fetal heartbeat auscultated as follows:
  - 10–12 weeks—heard with Doppler (rate 120–160 beats/min)
  - 17–20 weeks—heard with stethoscope

c. Fetal movement can be palpated by examiner at 20 weeks' gestation.

7. **Reflexes.** At least brachial and patellar assessed. Hyperreflexia could indicate developing PIH (see Procedure 3: Deep Tendon Reflexes and Clonus Assessment; PIH is discussed in Chapter 2).

8. **Pelvic exam.** External and internal genitals inspected, Pap obtained; gonorrhea culture (and sometimes chlamydia screen) obtained; changes of pregnancy noted, including Chadwick's sign, Goodell's sign. Uterine size evaluated to determine whether size seems appropriate for length of gestation. Ovaries palpated. Pelvic dimensions assessed to estimate whether pelvic size adequate for a vaginal birth.

The following dimensions are considered necessary for vaginal birth (See Figures 1–1 to 1–3):

- Pelvic inlet: Diagonal conjugate (extends from lower border of symphysis pubis to sacral promontory) at least 11.5 cm.
- Pelvic outlet: Anteroposterior diameter (from lower border of symphysis pubis to tip of sacrum) 9.5–11.5 cm.
- Pelvic outlet: Transverse diameter (measured by placing a fist between the ischial tuberosities) (Figure 1–2) 8–10 cm.
- Subpubic angle: Obtained by palpating bony structure externally, normally 85–90 degrees (Figure 1–3).
- Mobility of coccyx assessed by pressing on coccyx; it should be mobile.

9. **Rectal exam.** Rashes, lumps, hemorrhoids noted; woman with hemorrhoids should be assessed for problems with constipation.

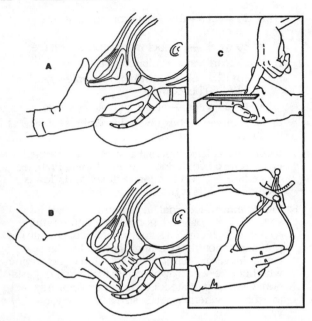

Figure 1–1   Manual measurement of inlet and outlet.
A, Estimation of diagonal conjugate, which extends
from the lower border of the symphysis pubis to the
sacral promontory. B, Estimation of anteroposterior
diameter of the outlet, which extends from the lower
border of the symphysis pubis to the tip of the sacrum.
C, Methods that may be used to check manual estima-
tion of anteroposterior measurements.

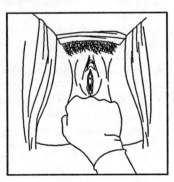

Figure 1–2   Use of
closed fist to measure
outlet. Most examiners
know the distance be-
tween the first and last
proximal knuckles.
If not, a measuring
device can be used.

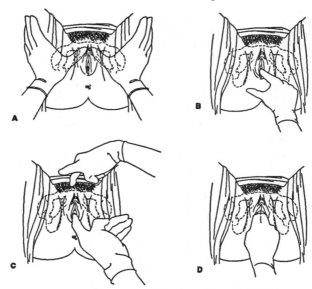

Figure 1–3 Evaluation of outlet. **A,** *Estimation of suprapubic angle.* **B,** *Estimation of length of pubic ramus.* **C,** *Estimation of depth and inclination of pubis.* **D,** *Estimation of contour of suprapubic angle.*

Determination of Due Date

The due date (date around which childbirth will occur) helps the care giver determine if the fetus is growing appropriately and whether the start of labor occurs at the correct time or prematurely. The due date, also called the EDB (estimated date of birth), EDD (estimated date of delivery), or EDC (estimated date of confinement) is calculated using a formula called Nägele's Rule. To use this formula one begins with the first day of the woman's last menstrual period (LMP), subtracts three months, and adds seven days. For example:

First day of LMP	November 21
Subtract 3 months	−3 months
	August 21
Add 7 days	+7 days
EDB	August 28

Due date can also be calculated using a gestational wheel. Some women do not have regular menstrual cycles or may not keep track of their menses. Thus, other methods are also used to date the pregnancy. These include the following:

1. **Uterine assessment, or sizing the uterus.**
   A skilled examiner can determine by bimanual examination if the size of the uterus is appropriate for the weeks of pregnancy. This is an especially valuable technique in the first trimester.

2. **Measurement of fundal height.** After the first trimester the uterus is palpable in the abdomen. Its height can be measured by using a centimeter tape measure to measure the distance from the top of the symphysis pubis to the top of the fundus. Fundal height corresponds well with weeks of gestation, especially between 20 and 31 weeks. For example, 24 cm would suggest 24 weeks' gestation.

3. **Quickening (perception of fetal movement by the mother).** This almost always occurs by 19 to 20 weeks' gestation. Because quickening may occur any time from 16 to 22 weeks, this is a less specific measure.

4. **Fetal heartbeat.** The heartbeat can be detected with a Doppler by 10–12 weeks' gestation and with a fetoscope by 19–20 weeks' gestation.

5. **Ultrasound.** This procedure can be used to detect a gestational sac in early pregnancy and to determine specific fetal measurements such as biparietal diameter. These measurements are useful in determining gestational age.

Frequency of Prenatal Visits in Normal Pregnancy

- Every four weeks for first 28 weeks of gestation
- Every two weeks to week 36
- After week 36, weekly until birth

Initial Psychosocial Assessment

The psychosocial assessment helps to determine the woman's attitude about the pregnancy, her teaching needs, the support systems she has available to her, her cultural or religious preferences, economic status, and living conditions. The following critical nursing assessments require further evaluation and intervention:

- Marked anxiety, apathy, fear, or anger about the pregnancy
- Isolated home environment without support systems available
- Language barriers
- Cultural practices that might endanger the child
- Long-term family problems
- Unstable or limited economic status; limited prenatal care
- Crowded or questionable living conditions

Regular Prenatal Visits

Critical nursing responsibilities

1. Weigh woman. During first trimester woman gains 3.5–5 lb; during second and third trimesters she gains about 1 lb/week. Thus, when she is seen every four weeks a 4-lb gain is normal.

   Be alert for:
   - Inadequate gain—evaluate reasons, counsel on nutrition
   - Excessive gain—often first sign of developing pregnancy-induced hypertension (PIH), a major complication of pregnancy (See Chapter 2 for further assessments.)

2. Vital signs. Pulse may increase slightly. BP usually decreases slightly toward midpregnancy and gradually returns to normal. Temperature and respirations may be omitted unless adverse symptoms are present.

   Be alert for:
   - Rapid pulse—could indicate anxiety or cardiac problem. Report findings
   - Elevated BP—a cardinal sign of PIH (See Chapter 2 for further assessments.)

3. Assess for edema. Some edema of ankles and feet is normal, especially in last trimester.

Be alert for:
- Edema of hands, face, and legs—usually related to weight gain and may indicate PIH (See Chapter 2 for further assessments.)

4. Dipstick urine specimen.

   Be alert for:
   - Proteinuria 1+. Could indicate PIH (See Chapter 2.)

   - Glycosuria—slight glycosuria may be normal but requires further assessment. Might indicate gestational diabetes mellitus (GDM) (See Chapter 2 for further assessments.)

5. Between 24–28 weeks' gestation a one-hour glucose screen is done. Plasma glucose levels > 140 mg/dL indicate GDM. Woman should be referred to physician.

6. Ask whether woman is experiencing any of the danger signs of pregnancy (see following discussion). Ask about the common discomforts of pregnancy and provide appropriate information (see pages 21–23).

Certified nurse-midwife, nurse practitioner, or physician completes remainder of exam, which includes:

1. Review of history and findings

2. Assessment of uterine size, measurement of fundal height

3. Assessment of fetal heartbeat (normal 120–160 bpm) and position

4. Assessment of deep tendon reflexes (DTRs), clonus (see Procedure 3: Deep Tendon Reflexes and Clonus Assessment)

5. Vaginal exam not repeated until last weeks of pregnancy

Danger Signs of Pregnancy and Their Possible Causes

Table 1–1 identifies the danger signs of pregnancy and their possible causes. These findings indicate a poten-

Table 1–1 Danger Signs in Pregnancy

The woman should report the following danger signs in pregnancy immediately:

Danger Sign	Possible Cause
1. Sudden gush of fluid from vagina	Premature rupture of membranes
2. Vaginal bleeding	Abruptio placentae, placenta previa, lesions of cervix or vagina, "bloody show"
3. Abdominal pain	Premature labor, abruptio placentae
4. Temperature above 38.3C (101F) and chills	Infection
5. Dizziness, blurring of vision, double vision, spots before eyes	Hypertension, preeclampsia
6. Persistent vomiting	Hyperemesis gravidarum
7. Severe headache	Hypertension, preeclampsia
8. Edema of hands, face, legs, and feet	Preeclampsia
9. Muscular irritability, convulsions	Preeclampsia, eclampsia
10. Epigastric pain	Preeclampsia-ischemia in major abdominal vessels
11. Oliguria	Renal impairment, decreased fluid intake
12. Dysuria	Urinary tract infection
13. Absence of fetal movement	Maternal medication, obesity, fetal death

tially serious problem and require further assessment. The nurse reviews these signs, and stresses to the woman the importance of reporting them immediately should they occur. **Discuss them at each prenatal visit.**

Essential Precautions in Practice

During Prenatal Examinations

Examples of times when gloves should be worn include the following:

- When drawing blood for lab work
- When handling urine specimens
- During pelvic examinations (sterile gloves)

In most instances in a clinic or office setting, gowns and goggles are not necessary because splashing of fluids is unlikely.

REMEMBER to wash your hands prior to putting the disposable gloves on and AGAIN immediately after you remove the gloves.

For further information consult OSHA and CDC guidelines.

PRENATAL NUTRITION

General Guidelines

1. Recommended dietary allowance (RDA) for most nutrients increases.
2. For a woman of normal prepregnant weight, the Institute of Medicine (1992) recommends a 25–35-lb gain.
3. Pattern of weight gain:
   - First trimester: 3.5–5 lb (1.6–2.3 kg.)
   - Second and third trimester: about 1 lb per week
   - Caloric increase: **only 300 kcal day.** Idea that woman is "eating for two" can lead to excessive weight gain
4. Overweight women should **not** diet during pregnancy.
5. In second and third trimesters, further evaluation indicated for the following:
   - Inadequate gain (less than 2.2 lb [1 kg]/month)
   - Excessive gain (more than 6.6 lb [3 kg]/month)

CRITICAL INFORMATION IN COUNSELING ABOUT NUTRITION

1. Stress the use of the Food Guide Pyramid, including the following:

   Bread, cereal, rice, and pasta: Adults need 6 to 11 servings (1 serving = 1 slice bread, 1 oz dry cereal, 1/2 hamburger roll, 1 tortilla, 1/2 cup pasta, 1/2 cup rice or grits).

   Vegetable group: Adults need 3 to 5 servings (1 serving = 1/2 cup cooked vegetables; 1 cup raw vegetables)

   Fruit group: Adults need 2 to 4 servings (1 serving = 1 medium-sized piece of fruit, 1/2 cup of juice). One serving should be a good source of vitamin C.

   Milk, yogurt, cheese group: Adults need 2 to 3 servings (1 serving = 1 cup milk or yogurt, 1.5 oz hard cheese, 2 cups cottage cheese, 1 cup pudding made with milk).

   Meat, poultry, fish, dry beans, eggs, and nuts group: Adults need 2 to 3 servings (1 serving = 2 oz cooked lean meat, poultry, or fish; 2 eggs; 1/2 cup cooked legumes [kidney, lima, garbanzo, or soy beans, split peas, etc]; 6 oz tofu; 2 oz nuts or seeds; 4 T peanut butter).

   Fats, oils, sweets: Use sparingly.

2. To increase diet by 300 kcal, woman should add 2 milk servings and 1 meat or alternate.

3. To get maximum benefit without additional calories, use low-fat dairy products, lean cuts of meat, low-fat cooking methods such as baking or broiling instead of frying, etc.

4. Limit extras that have little nutritional value and are high in sugar or fat, such as doughnuts, chips, candy, mayonnaise, etc.

Nutrition for the Pregnant Adolescent

If adolescent is less than four years post-menarche, her nutritional needs include the increase for pregnancy (300 kcal) plus the intake necessary for her anticipated weight gain developmentally during the year she is pregnant. Adolescent diets tend to be deficient in iron and calcium.

Iron supplements are used and iron-rich foods are encouraged (see following discussion of nutrition for the woman with anemia). Folic acid supplements are also given. If the adolescent is unwilling or unable to consume sufficient calcium, supplements may be necessary, usually 1200 mg daily.

Note: Many adolescents have a better diet than believed. Thus their eating patterns over several days, not simply one day, should be assessed.

Nutrition for the Pregnant Vegetarian

There are several types of vegetarians. Lacto-ovovegetarians include milk, dairy products, and eggs in their diet. Some also include fish and poultry. Lactovegetarians include dairy products but no eggs. Vegans are "pure" vegetarians who will not eat any food from animal sources.

If her diet permits, a woman can obtain adequate complete proteins from dairy products and eggs. Pure vegans must use complementing proteins such as unrefined grains (brown rice, whole wheat), legumes (beans, split peas, lentils), and nuts and seeds (in large quantities). Vegans should take a daily supplement of 4 gm of vitamin B_{12}. Vegetarian diets also tend to be low in iron and zinc and supplementation is often necessary.

Nutrition for the Woman with Anemia

To correct iron-deficiency anemia the woman will be given iron supplements. The nurse should explain to her that she can also help herself by the following dietary practices:

- Regularly eat meat, poultry, and fish, which are good sources of iron.
- Consume iron-fortified cereals and breads.
- Iron absorption is increased when vitamin C is taken with meals. Good sources of vitamin C include citrus fruits, strawberries, tomatoes, cantaloupe, broccoli, peppers, and potatoes.
- Select iron-rich vegetables such as spinach, broccoli, dandelion greens, and other green leafy vegetables.
- Use iron pots and pans for cooking.

RELIEF OF THE COMMON DISCOMFORTS OF PREGNANCY

Because of the physical and physiologic changes that occur during pregnancy, the woman may experience a variety of discomforts. The nurse has the primary responsibility for teaching the woman self-care measures to help alleviate these discomforts. The following section focuses on common discomforts and identifies interventions that may be effective:

First Trimester

Nausea and vomiting

- Avoid odors or factors that trigger nausea.
- Eat dry toast or crackers before arising.
- Have small but frequent dry meals with fluids between meals.
- Avoid greasy or highly seasoned foods.
- Drink carbonated beverages or herbal teas (peppermint, chamomile, spearmint, etc.).
- May benefit from acupressure wrist bands or acupressure to appropriate pressure points.

Urinary frequency

- Increase daytime fluid intake; void when the urge is felt.
- Decrease fluid **only** in the evening to decrease nocturia.

Breast tenderness

- Wear well-fitting, supportive bra.

Increased vaginal discharge

- Bathe daily but avoid douching, nylon panties, and pantyhose.
- Wear cotton underpants.

Nasal stuffiness and epistaxis

- May be unresponsive; cool air vaporizer may help.
- Avoid nasal sprays and decongestants.

Ptyalism

- Use astringent mouthwash, chew gum, suck hard candy.

Second and Third Trimesters

Pyrosis (heartburn)

- Eat small, frequent meals; avoid overeating or lying down afterward.
- Use low-sodium antacids, avoid sodium bicarbonate.

Ankle edema

- Dorsiflex foot frequently; elevate legs when sitting or resting.
- Avoid tight garters or constricting bands.

Varicose veins

- Wear supportive hose and elevate feet frequently.
- Avoid crossing legs at knees, prolonged standing, and garters.

Constipation

- Increase fluid in diet. (Drink at least eight 8-oz glasses daily.)
- Increase fiber. (Increase fruits/vegetables to six servings; choose fresh fruit when possible and include prunes or prune juice; increase grains to six servings and choose unrefined grains, such as whole wheat, brown rice and bran; include legumes in place of meat.)
- Increase daily exercise to promote peristalsis.

Hemorrhoids

- Avoid constipation and straining to defecate.
- Reinsert into rectum if necessary; treat with topical anesthetics, warm soaks or sitz baths, ice packs.

Backache

- Use good body mechanics; do pelvic tilt exercise regularly.
- Avoid uncomfortable working heights, high-heeled shoes, lifting heavy loads, and fatigue.

Leg cramps

- Practice dorsiflexing foot to stretch affected muscle.
- Apply heat to affected muscle.

Faintness

- Avoid prolonged standing in warm area; arise slowly from resting position.

Dyspnea

- Use proper posture when sitting or standing; sleep propped up with pillows if problem occurs at night.

Difficulty sleeping

- Drink a warm (caffeine-free) beverage before bed.
- Use pillows to provide support for back, between legs, or for upper arm when side-lying.

Flatulence

- Chew food thoroughly and avoid gas-forming food.
- Exercise regularly and maintain normal bowel habits.

Carpal tunnel syndrome

- Avoid aggravating hand movements; use splint as prescribed.
- Elevate affected arm.

PROMOTION OF SELF-CARE DURING PREGNANCY

Pregnant women may have questions about a variety of issues, which they will often raise with the prenatal nurse. The following discussion highlights critical information that the nurse should provide about selected topics.

Monitoring Fetal Activity

Vigorous fetal activity indicates fetal well-being, whereas a marked decrease in fetal activity may indicate fetal compromise and requires immediate evaluation. Fetal activity may be affected by drugs, cigarette smoking, sound, fetal sleep periods, blood glucose levels, and time of day. It has become accepted practice to teach pregnant women to monitor fetal activity daily beginning at about 27 weeks' gestation. Most healthy babies move at least ten times in 12 hours.

The woman begins counting fetal movements at a specified time twice daily, preferably about one hour after eating and while lying on her side. Movements are counted for 20–30 minutes; five to six movements in that time is considered reassuring. If there are fewer than three movements in that time the woman should continue counting for an hour or more. She should contact her care giver if there are fewer than ten movements in a 12-hour period OR no movements in the morning OR less than three fetal movements in eight hours. The care giver will probably order a nonstress test (NST). Alternately, the woman begins counting at a specified time daily and counts until ten fetal movements have occured. She should contact her care giver if there are fewer than ten movements in 3 hours or if it takes much longer each day to note ten movements.

Bathing

Daily bathing, by shower or in a tub, is important. The woman should take care to avoid slipping, especially because of her changed center of gravity. A rubber tub mat helps avoid this. **Stress that tub baths are contraindicated in the presence of ruptured membranes or vaginal bleeding to avoid introducing infection.**

Employment

Major problems with employment during pregnancy include exposure to fetotoxic hazards, excessive physical strain, overfatigue, medical or pregnancy-related complications, and, in later pregnancy, difficulty with occupations involving balance. Advise the woman who continues working to use breaks and lunch for rest, preferably on her side. Women who stand in place for long periods should dorsiflex their feet and walk around periodically to avoid problems with varicose veins, phlebitis, and edema.

Travel

If no complications exist, there are no restrictions on travel. Travel by plane or train is preferable for long distances. The woman should walk about periodically to avoid phlebitis. If traveling by car she should plan to stop every two hours and walk around for ten minutes. Seat belts should be worn with the lap belt positioned under the abdomen.

Exercise

The woman is encouraged to exercise at least three times/week. Swimming, cycling, walking, and cross-country skiing are good choices. In general, pregnancy is not the time to learn a new or strenuous sport. She should wear a supportive bra and appropriate shoes, should avoid hyperthermia, and should take fluids liberally to avoid dehydration. The woman should exercise for shorter intervals and should stop when she becomes fatigued. To avoid supine hypotensive syndrome she should avoid lying flat on her back to exercise after the first trimester. Dizziness, extreme shortness of breath, tingling and numbness, palpitations, abdominal pain, vaginal bleeding, and abrupt cessation of fetal movement should be reported to her care giver.
Stress the importance of adequate rest.

Exercises in Preparation for Childbirth

Teach abdominal tightening; partial, bent-knee sit-ups; Kegel exercises; and tailor sitting.

Sexual Activity

Change in desire is normal and may vary according to trimester. In the first trimester, fatigue, nausea, and breast tenderness may lead to decreased desire for some women. Other women experience no change. The second trimester may be a time of increased desire. The third trimester may lead to decreased desire. Woman should avoid lying flat on her back for intercourse after the fourth month to avoid vena caval syndrome. If that position is preferred she should place a pillow under her right hip to displace the uterus. Change in position, such as side-lying, female superior, or vaginal rear entry, may become necessary as her uterus enlarges. In the last weeks of pregnancy orgasms may be more intense and may be followed by uterine cramping.

Stress that sexual intercourse is contraindicated once the membranes are ruptured or in the presence of vaginal bleeding to avoid introducing infection. Women with a history of preterm labor may be advised to avoid intercourse in the third trimester because the oxytocin that is released with orgasm or with breast stimulation may trigger contractions. Couples who prefer anal intercourse should avoid going from anal penetration to vaginal penetration because of the risk of introducing infection.

Men may notice a change in their level of desire, too. If a man feels the desire for further sexual release he may need to masturbate, either with his partner or in private.

The couple can also be encouraged to explore other methods of expressing intimacy and affection, such as stroking, cuddling, and kissing.

Medications, Alcohol, Smoking

Women should avoid taking medication when pregnant—both prescribed and over-the-counter medication. If the need for medication arises, the woman should make certain her care giver knows that she is pregnant. Smoking is related to lower birth weight infants and to preterm labor. Women should avoid it as much as possible. Alcohol has been linked to neurologic deficits in newborns and to low birth weight. Heavy drinking may lead to fetal alcohol syndrome. Since it is not clear how much alcohol is problematic it should be avoided. Similarly women should avoid cocaine, crack, marijuana, and all social and street drugs during pregnancy.

CHARTING

Most prenatal records are composed of a series of columns for making notations succinctly. These columns include height, weight, blood pressure, urine, fetal heart rate, fundal height, edema, fetal movement, clonus, etc. Notations should be made in the "comments" about any deviations from normal, about any teaching that is done, and about any special procedures. Charting on the prenatal record tends to be especially succinct, as the following example demonstrates:

> Basic four food groups and caloric increases for pregnancy discussed. Handout on prenatal nutrition reviewed and given to client. Reports she is taking prenatal vitamins regularly. States that nausea has decreased and she is walking 2 miles/four times/week. No problems or distress. Will call if symptoms develop. A. Smythe, RN

ASSESSMENT OF FETAL WELL-BEING

Ultrasound

Obstetric ultrasound is done either vaginally or transabdominally depending on the timing in pregnancy and the purpose of the ultrasound. Ultrasound is generally painless and nonradiating to the woman and fetus; it has no known harmful effects. Serial studies can be done for assessment and comparison.

Ultrasound can be used for early identification of pregnancy (as early as 5th–6th week after LMP); for identification of more than one fetus; to measure biparietal diameter; to detect fetal anomalies, hydramnios (excess amniotic fluid) or oligohydramnios (too little fluid); to locate and grade the placenta; to observe fetal heart rate, movement, respirations, position and presentation, or fetal death.

Nursing interventions The nurse provides an opportunity for the woman to ask questions and acts as a client advocate.

Nonstress Test

The nonstress test (NST) is used to assess fetal status using an electronic fetal monitor to observe baseline variability and acceleration of fetal heart rate (FHR) with movement. FHR accelerations indicate that the fetal central and autonomic nervous systems have not been affected by decreased oxygen to the fetus.

Procedure   NST may be done in a clinic or an inpatient setting. The woman is placed in semi-Fowler's position, in a side-lying position, or in a reclining chair. Two belts are placed on the woman's abdomen: one records the FHR, the other records uterine or fetal movement. The fetal monitor begins recording activity. The woman is instructed to press a button on the monitor (or on the uterine belt) each time she feels the fetus move. This causes a mark on the tracing paper. An assessment can then be made as to whether FHR accelerations occurred with each fetal movement.

Interpretation of NST Results

- **Reactive test** shows at least two accelerations of FHR with fetal movements, of 15 beats/min, lasting 15 seconds or more, over a period of 20 minutes (Figure 1–4).
- **Nonreactive test** is one in which the reactive criteria are not met (Figure 1–5).
- **Unsatisfactory test** is one in which data cannot be interpreted or there is inadequate fetal activity.

A reactive NST usually indicates fetal well-being and the test does not need to be repeated for a week. A nonreactive NST indicates the need for further testing.

Nursing interventions   The nurse explains the procedure, administers the NST, interprets the results, and reports the findings to the physician/certified nurse-midwife. If the fetus is not moving well, it is sometimes helpful to have the mother drink a glass of juice to increase her blood glucose level. This seems to result in increased fetal activity.

Note: If any decelerations in FHR occur during the procedure, the physician/nurse-midwife should be notified for further evaluation of fetal status.

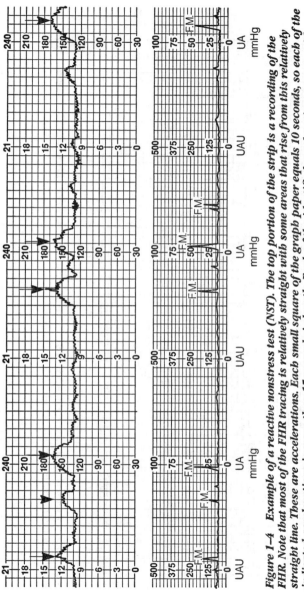

Figure 1–4   Example of a reactive nonstress test (NST). The top portion of the strip is a recording of the FHR. Note that most of the FHR tracing is relatively straight with some areas that rise from this relatively straight line. These are accelerations. Each small square of the graph paper equals 10 seconds, so each of the indicated accelerations is more than 15 seconds in length. Each of the identified accelerations occurs with a fetal movement (FM), which is recorded on the bottom portion of the strip. The criteria for a reactive NST have been met on this tracing.

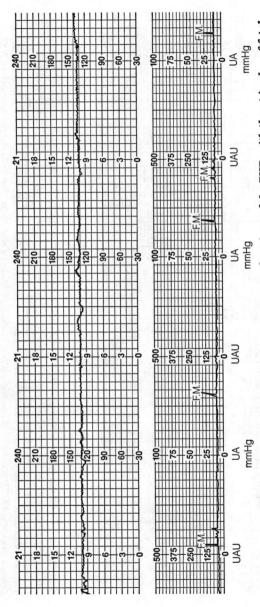

Figure 1–5   Example of a nonreactive NST. There are no accelerations of the FHR, with the episodes of fetal movement indicated on the bottom portion of the strip.

Biophysical Profile (BBP)

The biophysical profile is a collection of information regarding selected fetal measurements and assessments of the fetus and the amniotic fluid. It includes five variables: fetal breathing movements, body movement, tone, FHR activity, and amniotic fluid volume. Table 1–2 identifies scoring techniques and interpretation. Table 1–3 outlines a management protocol.

Amniotic Fluid Analysis (Amniocentesis)

Amniotic fluid can be withdrawn through a needle inserted through the abdominal wall into the uterus and analyzed to obtain valuable information about fetal status. Amniotic fluid analysis provides genetic information about the fetus and can also be used to determine fetal lung maturity. (See Procedure 1: Amniocentesis: Nursing Responsibilities.)

Fetal lung maturity can be ascertained by determining the ratio of the phospholipids, lecithin and sphingomyelin. These are two components of surfactant, the substance that lowers the surface tension of the alveoli of the lungs when the newborn exhales, thereby preventing lung collapse. Early in pregnancy the sphingomyelin component is greater than the lecithin so that the lecithin to sphingomyelin (L/S) ratio is low. As pregnancy progresses the lecithin increases. Fetal maturity is indicated by an L/S ratio of 2:1 or greater. **Note: delayed lung maturation is often seen in infants born to diabetic mothers. Thus an L/S ratio of 3:1 or higher may be necessary in these infants to ensure lung maturity.**

Another phospholipid, phosphatidylglycerol (PG), appears in the amniotic fluid after about 35 weeks' gestation and the amount continues to increase to term.

Amniotic creatinine progressively increases with the length of pregnancy, apparently because of increasing fetal muscle mass and maturing fetal renal function. Creatinine levels of 2 mg/dL are associated with fetal maturity.

In summary, fetal lung maturity is probable if the following are present:

- L/S ratio of 2:1 or greater
- PG present
- Amniotic creatinine of 2 mg/dL

Table 1–2   Biophysical Profile Scoring: Technique and Interpretation

Biophysical Variable	Normal (Score = 2)	Abnormal (Score = 0)
1. Fetal breathing movements	≥ episode of ≥30 sec in 30 min	Absent or no episode of ≥30 sec in 30 min
2. Gross body movements	≥ 3 discrete body/limb movements in 30 min (episodes of active continuous movement considered as single movement)	≤ 2 episodes of body/limb movements in 30 min
3. Fetal tone	≥ 1 episode of active extension with return to flexion of fetal limb(s) or trunk. Opening and closing of hand considered normal tone	Either slow extension with return to partial extension or movement of limb in full extension or absent fetal movement
4. Reactive fetal heart rate	≥ 2 episodes of acceleration of ≥15 bpm and of ≥ 15 sec associated with fetal movement in 20 min	< 2 episodes of acceleration of fetal heart rate or acceleration of <15 bpm in 20 min
5. Qualitative amniotic fluid volume	≥ 1 pocket of fluid measuring ≥ 1 cm in two perpendicular planes	Either no pockets or a pocket <1 cm in two perpendicular planes

Source: Manning FA et al: Fetal assessment based on fetal biophysical profile scoring: Experience in 12,620 referred high-risk pregnancies. *Am J Obstet Gynecol* 1985; 151(3): 344.

Table 1–3 Management Based on Biophysical Profile Score*

Attained Score	Intervention
10 of 10, or 8 of 10, with normal amniotic fluid volume.	No intervention needed, normal finding.
8 of 10 with abnormal amniotic fluid volume	If fetal renal function is normal and membranes are intact, delivery is indicated.
6 of 10 with normal amniotic fluid volume.	Deliver fetus if it is mature. If immature, repeat test within 24 hours. If score is 6 of 10 or below, deliver fetus.
4 of 10, or 2 of 10, or 1 of 10.	Deliver fetus.

*Adapted from Manning FA: The biophysical profile: Contemporary use. Tenth International Symposium on Perinatal Medicine and Obstetrical Ultrasound, April 9–12, 1990, Las Vegas, Nevada.

REFERENCES

Blackburn ST, Loper DL: *Maternal, Fetal, and Neonatal Physiology: A Clinical Perspective*. Philadelphia: Saunders, 1992.

Institute of Medicine, Subcommittee for a Clinical Application Guide: *Nutrition during Pregnancy and Lactation: An Implementation Guide*. Washington DC: National Academy Press, 1992.

Rubin R: *Maternal Identity and the Maternal Experience*. New York: Springer, 1984.

CHAPTER 2

The At-Risk Antepartal Client

DIABETES MELLITUS

Overview

In diabetes mellitus the pancreas does not produce enough insulin to allow necessary carbohydrate metabolism. Glucose does not enter the cells, and they become energy depleted. The physiologic changes of pregnancy can drastically alter insulin requirements. In the first half of pregnancy maternal hormones stimulate increased insulin production by the pancreas and increased tissue response to insulin. In the second half of pregnancy maternal hormones cause increased resistance to insulin. Concurrently, increased amounts of maternal glucose are being diverted to the fetus. Any diabetic potential may be influenced by this increased stress on the β-cells of the pancreas. **Gestational diabetes mellitus (GDM)** refers to diabetes that develops during pregnancy, often in the third trimester. To detect this condition, most women are screened for GDM between 24 and 28 weeks' gestation, using a 50-gram, 1-hour oral glucose screen. Often gestational diabetes can be managed with diet, although some women will receive regular insulin as well.

For women with **pregestational diabetes mellitus** (DM present before conception), the changes in glucose metabolism that result with pregnancy can affect diabetic control and can contribute to possible accelerations of the vascular disease associated with DM. The infant of a diabetic mother (IDM) is at greater risk for mortality or morbidity.

Pregestational diabetes can be type I (insulin dependent) or type II (non–insulin-dependent). Women with pregestational DM are treated with insulin only because oral anti-hyperglycemic agents are teratogenic to the fetus.

Maternal risks with diabetic pregnancy include the following: hydramnios (excessive volume of amniotic fluid), pregnancy-induced hypertension, ketoacidosis, fetal macrosomia leading to dystocia (difficult labor), anemia, monilial vaginitis, urinary tract infection (UTI), and retinopathy.

Fetal-neonatal risks include the following: intrauterine growth retardation (IUGR), macrosomia (large-size infant), hypoglycemia, respiratory distress syndrome, hyperbilirubinemia, and congenital anomalies.

Medical Management

1. **Dietary regulation.** Caloric needs of pregnant women are not altered by diabetes. They need 30 kcal/kg ideal body weight (IBW) during first trimester and 35–36 kcal/kg IBW during second and third trimesters. Fifty to sixty percent of calories should come from complex carbohydrates, 12% to 20% from protein, and 20% to 30% from fat. This is divided among three meals and three snacks. Prebedtime snack is most important because of risk of hypoglycemia during the night and should contain both protein and complex carbohydrates.

2. **Glucose monitoring.** Urine monitoring is seldom used. Many physicians have women come in weekly for assessment of fasting glucose levels and periodic postprandial levels. Most also have the woman do home monitoring of blood glucose levels QID— a fasting level before breakfast and then two hours after each meal. Optimal range, fasting: 60–100 mg/dL, two hours postprandial: 100–140 mg/dL (Ratner 1993).

3. **Insulin administration.** The dosage of human insulin is generally divided as follows: 2/3 of total dose taken in am with a 2:1 ratio of intermediate insulin to regular; remaining 1/3 of dose taken with evening meal in a ratio of 1:1. The amount of insulin needed usually increases during each trimester of pregnancy.
   Note: oral hypoglycemics are teratogenic and are never used in pregnancy.

4. **Evaluation of fetal status.** Woman is taught to monitor daily fetal activity (Chapter 1). Nonstress

tests (NSTs) (see Chapter 1) are begun weekly at 28 weeks and increase to twice weekly at 32 weeks (Landon & Gable 1991). Ultrasounds are done at 18 weeks and 28 weeks to establish gestational age and assess for intrauterine growth retardation; biophysical profiles are done in third trimester to evaluate fetal well-being.

Critical Nursing Assessments

1. Assess urine for glucose and ketones at each prenatal visit.

2. Assess results of blood glucose testing for women with diagnosed GDM or pregestational DM.

3. Assess for any signs of UTI (dysuria, urgency, frequency, hematuria) or monilial vaginitis (excessive itching, curdy white discharge, dyspareunia).

4. Assess woman's understanding of her condition, its treatment, and implications.
   Be alert for: hyperglycemia, hypoglycemia, evidence of infection, signs of vascular complications (ulceration of extremities, visual changes, and so forth).

Sample Nursing Diagnoses

1. Knowledge deficit related to lack of information about the disease and its implications for the woman and her unborn child.

2. Altered family processes related to the client's hospitalization for stabilization of her DM.

Critical Nursing Interventions

1. Obtain serum glucose readings at the specified times (if woman is hospitalized).

2. Administer insulin as prescribed. Have a second nurse verify the dosage before administering the insulin.

3. Hypoglycemia may be caused by too much insulin or too little food. Typically the onset is sudden (minutes to 1/2 hour). Monitor for signs of developing

hypoglycemia including sweating, periodic tingling, disorientation, shakiness, pallor, clammy skin, irritability, hunger, headache, blurred vision, and, if untreated, convulsions and coma. If they occur, immediately check woman's capillary glucose level (and teach her to do the same following discharge). Follow agency policy regarding procedure for correcting hypoglycemia for blood glucose < 60 mg/dL. This may include 15-oz milk or 12-oz orange juice (Mandeville & Troiano, 1992). If woman is not alert enough to swallow, give 1 mg glucagon subq or IM and notify physician.

4. Hyperglycemia is generally caused by too much food and too little insulin, and typically the onset is slow (days). Observe for signs of developing hyperglycemia such as polyuria, polydipsia, dry mouth, increased appetite, fatigue, nausea, hot and flushed skin, rapid and deep breathing, abdominal cramps, acetone breath, headache, drowsiness, depressed reflexes, oliguria or anuria, and stupor or coma. If hyperglycemia is suspected, obtain frequent measures of blood glucose; check urine for acetone. Administer prescribed amount of regular insulin subcutaneously, intravenously, or by a combination of routes. Replace fluids; measure I & O.

5. Monitor fetal status including fetal heart rate (FHR) q4h; assist woman with determining fetal movement record daily; do NSTs as ordered while woman is hospitalized.

6. Provide appropriate American Diabetes Association (ADA) diet as indicated. Work with dietitian to ensure appropriate teaching is provided for the woman.

7. Complete client teaching about the following:

   • Procedure for home monitoring of blood glucose: Wash hands thoroughly before finger puncture. Sides of fingers should be punctured (ends contain more pain sensitive nerves). Hanging arm down for 30 sec before puncture increases blood flow to fingers. Spring-loaded devices are available to make puncture easier. Cleanse finger with alcohol pad first and allow alcohol to air dry. Touch blood droplet, not finger, to test pad on strip. Droplet should completely cover the test pad. If using visual method, wait prescribed time and compare color to color chart. If using a glucose meter, follow directions for use exactly. Record results and bring record sheet to each prenatal visit.

- Procedure for insulin administration (if woman is not already familiar with it).
- Signs of hypoglycemia and required treatment.
- Signs of hyperglycemia and required treatment.
- ADA diet.

8. Review the following critical aspects of the care you have provided:

   - Have I administered the correct doses of insulin at the specified times after first determining blood glucose levels?

Essential Precautions in Practice

A Pregnant Woman with Diabetes Mellitus

In caring for a pregnant woman with diabetes mellitus all the precautions apply that are established for any hospitalized pregnant, laboring, or postpartal woman. In addition, remember the following specifics:

- Wear gloves when doing fingersticks for glucose levels, when starting IVs, when testing urine for ketones, or when drawing blood for other laboratory tests.
- When teaching a woman to do her own blood glucose testing, gloves should be available and put on if it becomes necessary for the nurse to help the woman obtain a blood sample. The woman does not need to wear gloves during the procedure.
- Dispose of needles, syringes, lancets, and other sharp objects in appropriately labeled containers.

REMEMBER to wash your hands prior to putting the disposable gloves on and AGAIN immediately after you remove the gloves.

For further information consult OSHA and CDC guidelines.

- Have I been alert for any signs of hypoglycemia or hyperglycemia?
- Have I monitored FHR and fetal activity carefully and discussed with the woman her perceptions of fetal activity?
- Have I assessed the woman's understanding of her DM and answered her questions? Have I given her opportunities to practice specific skills as necessary?
- Have I ensured that the woman is eating the appropriate meals?

Evaluation

- The woman is able to discuss her condition and its possible impact on her pregnancy.
- The woman participates in developing a health-care regimen to meet her needs and follows it throughout pregnancy.
- The woman avoids developing hypoglycemia or hyperglycemia; if it does develop, therapy is successful in correcting it without complications.
- The woman gives birth to a healthy newborn.

PREGNANCY-INDUCED HYPERTENSION (PIH)

Overview

Pregnancy-induced hypertension (PIH), the most common hypertensive disorder in pregnancy, is characterized by the development of hypertension, proteinuria, and edema. The definition of PIH is a blood pressure (BP) of 140/90 mm Hg during the second half of pregnancy in a previously normotensive woman. An increase in systolic blood pressure of 30 mm Hg and/or of diastolic of 15 mm Hg over baseline also defines PIH. These blood pressure changes must be noted on at least two occasions six hours or more apart for the diagnosis to be made.

Mild preeclampsia is characterized by a BP of 140/90 or +30/+15 over baseline on two occasions at least five hours apart; generalized edema of the face, hands, legs, and ankles, which is usually associated with a weight gain of more than 1 lb/week; and proteinuria of 1+ to 2+ on dipstick (less than 5 gm in 24 hours).

Severe preeclampsia is characterized by a blood pressure of 160/110 on two occasions at least six hours apart while the woman is on bed rest; proteinuria > 5 gm in 24 hours (3+ to 4+ dipstick); oliguria (urine output < 400 mL/24 hr); headache, blurred vision, scotomata (spots before the eyes), and retinal edema on funduscopy (retinas appear wet and glistening); pulmonary edema; hyperreflexia; irritability; and epigastric pain.

Eclampsia is characterized by a grand mal seizure, which may be preceded by an elevated temperature as high as 38.4C (101F), or the temperature may remain normal. The woman may have just one seizure or from 2 to 20 or more. Symptoms may increase in severity: BP of 180/110 or higher, 4+ proteinuria, oliguria or anuria, and increased neurologic symptoms such as decreased sensorium or coma.

Maternal risks with PIH include the following: retinal detachment, central nervous system changes including hyperreflexia and seizure, HELLP syndrome (**h**emolysis, **e**levated **l**iver enzymes, and **l**ow **p**latelet count). Women who experience HELLP, a multiple organ failure syndrome, and their offspring have high morbidity and mortality rates.

Fetal-neonatal risks include the following: prematurity, intrauterine growth retardation, oversedation at birth because of maternal medications, and mortality rates of 10% with preeclampsia and 20% with eclampsia.

Medical Management

Mild preeclampsia (may be managed on outpatient basis in some cases):

1. **Promotion of good placental and renal perfusion.** Frequent rest periods are necessary during the day in a side-lying position. Specific guidelines regarding rest periods may be given, including the amount of time in each rest period, number of rest periods daily, and the activities during the day that are advisable or should be avoided. The more specific the guidelines, the more likely that the woman will clearly understand the information and restrictions.

2. **Dietary modifications.** Diet should be high in protein (80–100 gm/day, or 1.5 gm/kg/day). Sodium intake should be moderate, not exceeding 6 gm/day.

3. **Evaluation of fetal status.** NSTs and/or fetal biophysical profile are done on a weekly basis. Additional tests include serial ultrasounds to evaluate fetal growth, amniocentesis to determine fetal lung maturity, and a contraction stress test if nonstress test results indicate a need.

4. **Evaluation of maternal well-being.** The woman is seen every one to two weeks, is taught signs of a worsening condition, and does home blood pressure monitoring daily.

Severe Preeclampsia (hospitalization necessary):

1. **Promotion of maternal well-being.** Complete bed rest in left lateral position, which decreases pressure on vena cava, thereby increasing venous perfusion. Improved renal blood flow helps decrease angiotensin II levels, promotes diuresis, and lowers blood pressure. High protein, moderate sodium diet is continued. The woman is weighed daily (to detect edema) and evaluated for evidence of a change in condition through assessment of BP, TPR, deep tendon reflexes (DTRs) and clonus, edema (generalized and pitting), presence of headache, visual disturbances, and epigastric pain.

2. **Evaluation of laboratory data.** Daily hematocrit (rising value may be associated with decreasing vascular volume), daily liver enzyme testing including SGOT, SGPT, and LDH (a rise in these tests correlates with a worsening condition), daily uric acid and BUN (reflect renal status), platelet counts every two to three days if over $100,000/mm^3$, daily if under $100,000/mm^3$. (Platelet count may be included in preeclamptic or disseminated intravascular coagulation [DIC] screen, which also determines prothrombin time, partial thromboplastin time, fibrinogen and fibrin split products.) Platelet transfusions are indicated if the platelet count is below $20,000/mm^3$.

3. **Medication therapy.** Magnesium sulfate is the treatment of choice for preventing convulsion (see

Drug Guide 3: Magnesium Sulfate). Sedation with phenobarbital 30–60 mg p.o. q6h may be indicated. (Some physicians prefer diazepam [Valium].) An antihypertensive such as methyldopa (Aldomet), labetalol (Normodyne), or nifedipine (Procardia) may be used if the diastolic pressure is 110 mm Hg or above. Fluid and electrolytes are replaced as necessary based on the status of the woman.

Eclampsia

1. **Promotion of maternal well-being.** The therapies discussed previously are continued. Additional magnesium sulfate or sedation is used to stop the convulsion. The airway is maintained and the woman is monitored for pulmonary edema, which may be treated with furosemide (Lasix). Digitalis may be given for circulatory failure. The woman may be transferred to an intensive care unit.

Critical Nursing Assessments

1. Assess BP, pulse, and respirations q2–4h.

2. Assess temperature q4h unless elevated, then q2h.

3. Assess FHR when maternal vital signs (VS) are assessed or continuously with an electronic fetal monitor.

4. Assess intake and urinary output hourly or q4h. Output should be 700 mL/24 hr, or at least 30 mL/hr.

5. Assess urinary protein by dipstick of each urine specimen or a specimen from indwelling bladder catheter. **Assessment technique:** A small sample of urine is collected in a urine specimen bottle or in a syringe. A few drops of urine are placed on the treated section of the dipstick. The color of the treated urine is compared to samples on the dipstick container after a specified period of time. See dipstick container for specific instructions.

6. Assess urine specific gravity.

7. Assess for evidence of edema. **Assessment technique:** Assess for pitting edema by pressing over bony areas, usually over the shin. After pressing with one fingertip for three to five

seconds, evaluate the resulting depression. A slight depression is 1+, a pit one-inch deep is 4+.

8. Assess daily weight. Use the same scales each day, weigh at the same time each day with the woman in similar clothing.

9. Assess DTRs. Assess for clonus. (See Procedure 3: Deep Tendon Reflexes and Clonus Assessment.)

10. Assess breath sounds—rales will be heard if pulmonary edema is developing.

11. Assess laboratory results.

12. Assess woman's coping responses, level of understanding regarding her condition, and emotional status.

13. See Drug Guide 3: Magnesium Sulfate for specific nursing assessments during $MgSO_4$ therapy. **Be alert for:** Signs of worsening condition (increasing BP, headache, scotomata, increasing edema especially of hands and face, disorientation, epigastric pain, pitting edema); signs of $MgSO_4$ toxicity (respirations < 12–14/min, diminished or absent reflexes, urine output < 100 mL in four-hour period).

Sample Nursing Diagnoses

- Fluid volume deficit related to fluid shift from intravascular to extravascular space secondary to vasospasm.
- Risk for injury related to possibility of convulsion secondary to cerebral vasospasm or edema.
- Knowledge deficit related to lack of information about PIH and its implications for the woman and her unborn child.

Critical Nursing Interventions

If the woman is managed at home:

1. Teach the woman and her support person how to assess BP. Include positioning and specifics of the procedure. Assist them in developing a chart to record the findings. Instruct them about findings that should be reported to the physician.

2. Provide teaching about the rest period regimen. Explain the purpose of the side-lying position.

If the woman is hospitalized:

1. Monitor maternal BP, pulse and respirations, DTRs and clonus, and FHR q2–4h. Monitor oral temperature q4h unless elevated, then q2h. Weigh daily.

2. Monitor intake and output; monitor urine for proteinuria and specific gravity with each voiding or hourly if an indwelling catheter is in place. Output should be at least 30 mL/hr. Specific gravity of readings > 1.040 indicate oliguria.

3. Monitor for signs of worsening condition including headache, visual disturbances, epigastric pain, and change in level of consciousness at least q4h.

Essential Precautions in Practice

A Woman with PIH

In caring for a woman with PIH, all the precautions established for any hospitalized pregnant, laboring, or postpartal woman apply. In addition remember the following specifics:

- Wear gloves when testing urine for proteinuria, when starting IV for $MgSO_4$ therapy, when doing fingersticks to test hematocrit, or when drawing blood for other laboratory tests.
- If eclampsia occurs and the woman convulses, wear gloves when removing the airway.
- If incontinence occurs during the convulsion, wear a splash apron and gloves when cleansing the woman and while changing the bedding.
- Dispose of needles, syringes, lancets, and other sharp objects in appropriately labeled containers.

REMEMBER to wash your hands prior to putting disposable gloves on and AGAIN immediately after you remove the gloves.

For further information, consult OSHA and CDC guidelines.

4. Maintain woman in a side-lying position.

5. Provide emotional support and teaching regarding condition and treatment plan.

6. Administer $MgSO_4$ and other medications as ordered. Monitor for evidence of effectiveness or toxicity.

7. Provide a quiet, restful environment with limited visitors.

8. Pad side rails and take seizure precautions.

9. Review the following aspects of the care you have provided:

   • What is the woman's response to the medications? Am I seeing any potential side effects?

   • Is there a change in her ability to talk? Does she seem more irritable? Confused?

   • Is she complaining of headache or other symptoms that indicate a worsening condition?

   • Is the baby moving as much? Is FHR in normal range (120–160 beats/min)?

   • Positioning on which side produces the best results in fetal heart rate? Urine output? What can I do to help her maintain that position? A back rub? Pillows?

   • Have I taken necessary safety precautions, including padded side rails, quiet environment, calcium gluconate (magnesium sulfate antagonist) available?

Sample Nurse's Charting

4:00 pm BP stable at 142/96, P 88, R 18, T 98.4F. FHR 138. Lungs clear to auscultation. DTRs, patellar and brachial, 2+ with no clonus. Pitting edema 1+ in legs, some swelling of fingers—rings snug. Slight periorbital edema evident. Urine S.G. 1.034; hourly output 40 mL/hr through Foley. 2+ proteinuria. $MgSO_4$ maintenance dose running at 2 gm/hr per infusion pump. No edema, redness, or c/o discomfort at infusion site. Continuous EFM with FHR baseline 140–146, LTV average, STV present. Accelerations of 20 bpm for 20 sec noted with fetal movement. No decelerations noted. Client alert, responsive, oriented. States she has a slight headache but denies epigastric pain or visual changes. Resting quietly on her L side. Side rails padded and up. A. Smythe, RN

Evaluation

- The woman is able to explain PIH, its implications for her pregnancy, the treatment regimen, and possible complications.
- The woman does not have any eclamptic convulsions.
- The woman and her care givers detect any evidence of increasing severity of the PIH or possible complications early so that appropriate treatment measures can be instituted.
- The woman gives birth to a healthy newborn.

PRETERM LABOR

Overview

Labor that occurs between 20 and 37 completed weeks of gestation is referred to as *preterm labor.* It may result from maternal factors such as cardiovascular or renal disease, PIH, diabetes, abdominal surgery during pregnancy, a blow to the abdomen, uterine anomalies, cervical incompetence, DES exposure, history of cone biopsy, and maternal infection. Fetal factors include multiple pregnancy, hydramnios, and fetal infection, and placental factors include placenta previa and placenta abruptio.

The major maternal risks involve psychologic stress related to the woman's concern for her unborn child and physiologic side effects of the drugs used to stop labor. Fetal-neonatal risks are those related to the effects of prematurity.

Medical Management

1. **Confirmation of diagnosis.** A diagnosis of preterm labor is made if the gestation is between 20 and 37 weeks, if there are documented uterine contractions (four in 20 minutes or eight in 60 minutes), and ruptured membranes. If the membranes are not ruptured one of the following must be present: 80% cervical effacement, documented cervical changes, or 2 cm dilatation.

2. **Initial treatment.** Any medical conditions that may contribute to preterm labor should be treated. Mild

symptoms may be treated with bed rest and hydration per infusion. If labor continues or if symptoms are severe, tocolysis (use of medication to stop labor) is begun.

3. **Tocolysis.** Tocolytics currently used to arrest preterm labor include β-adrenergic agents and magnesium sulfate. The β-adrenergics used include ritodrine (Yutopar), which is FDA approved, and terbutaline (Brethine), which is not FDA approved for use in preterm labor but has become increasingly popular because it is effective and less expensive than ritodrine. If uterine contractions are mild, terbutaline is administered subcutaneously. With more pronounced contractions (or if subcutaneous terbutaline is not effective) terbutaline is administered intravenously until uterine activity ceases. The medication is then administered orally for long-term maintenance. Some facilities are also using a subcutaneous terbutaline pump for long-term tocolysis.

   Magnesium sulfate is also effective and has fewer side effects than the β-adrenergics. Six gm is administered IV over 30 min. A maintenance dose of 2–4 gm/hr via infusion pump is then used until contractions cease. Maternal serum level of 6–8 mg/dL is the effective range for tocolysis (Parsons & Spellacy 1994). (See Drug Guide 3: Magnesium Sulfate.) Long-term oral therapy may be accomplished with magnesium chloride, magnesium oxide, or magnesium gluconate at a dose of 250–450 mg q3hr.

4. Women who are at risk for preterm labor may benefit from participating in an at home preterm birth prevention program. Examples of major risk factors include a history of preterm labor, multiple gestation, uterine anomaly, DES exposure, hydramnios, two or more second trimester abortions, and uterine irritability.

Critical Nursing Assessments

1. Assess carefully for evidence of complications or side effects from tocolysis. These include tachycardia, palpitations, nervousness, nausea and vomiting, headache, hypotension.

Be alert for: evidence of pulmonary edema, the most serious complication. Signs include shortness of breath, chest tightness, dyspnea, rales, and rhonchi.

2. Assess for symptoms of magnesium toxicity in women receiving magnesium sulfate, including respirations < 12 min, diminished or absent DTRs, urine output < 100 mL in four-hour period.

Sample Nursing Diagnoses

- Knowledge deficit related to lack of information about causes, identification, and treatment of preterm labor.
- Fear related to the risks of early labor and birth.

Critical Nursing Interventions

Home care

1. Instruct women at risk about the signs and symptoms of preterm labor, which include the following:

   - Uterine contractions occurring q10min or more frequently
   - Mild menstrual-like cramps felt low in the abdomen or abdominal cramping with or without diarrhea
   - Feelings of pelvic pressure that may feel like the baby pressing down. The pressure may be constant or intermittent
   - Constant or intermittent low backache
   - A sudden change in vaginal discharge (an increase in amount, or a change to more clear and watery, or a pinkish tinge)

2. Instruct women on a home monitoring program that they will use a home uterine activity monitor to record and transmit uterine contractile activity via the phone once or twice daily to a nurse specially trained in assessing the signs and symptoms of preterm labor. The nurse uses the data received and the woman's reports of symptoms to evaluate the risk of preterm labor on a daily basis.

3. Teach the at-risk woman who is **not** on a preterm home monitoring program to evaluate contraction activity once or twice daily. Instruct her to lie on her side and place her fingertips on the fundus of the uterus. She checks for contractions (hardening of the fundus) for about one hour. Occasional contractions are probably normal Braxton Hicks contractions.

4. If the woman experiences contractions every ten minutes or any of the previously identified signs of labor, instruct her to do the following:

   - Empty her bladder and lie down, preferably on her left side.
   - Drink three to four 8-oz cups of fluid.
   - Palpate for uterine contractions.
   - Rest for 30 minutes after symptoms have subsided and gradually resume activity.
   - Call her health care provider if symptoms persist, even if uterine contractions are not palpable.

Hospital care

1. Promote bed rest in a side-lying position as much as possible.

2. Monitor BP, pulse, and respirations as ordered, especially when on tocolytic therapy.

3. Maintain continuous electronic monitoring of FHR and uterine contractions if ordered (see Chapter 3) and evaluate results.

4. Monitor intake and output.

5. Keep vaginal exams to a minimum.

6. Explain procedures to the woman and her partner; answer questions and provide emotional support.

7. Review the following critical aspects of the care you have provided:

   - What is the woman's response to the tocolysis? Is she showing any side effects of the medication?
   - Is she still having contractions? Have they increased or lessened? Is she showing other signs of labor?
   - What is the fetus' response?

- What position is most effective? Are there nursing measures I can use to help her tolerate the side-lying position and the effects of tocolysis?
- How is she coping emotionally? Have I spent enough time helping her to cope with the stress of the situation?

Sample Nurse's Charting
for Woman Receiving Subcutaneous Terbutaline

10:00 am BP stable at 108/70, P 104 and regular, R 18, T 98.0. FHR baseline 148–152, STV present, LTV average. No decelerations noted. No contractions for past 4 hr. Receiving subq terbutaline. Lungs clear to auscultation. c/o mild headache, relieved with Tylenol. IV infusing (see IV sheet). Voided 250 mL clear urine. Resting on L side. A. Smythe, RN

Evaluation

- The woman is able to discuss the cause, identification, and treatment of preterm labor.
- The woman understands self-care measures and can identify characteristics that should be reported to her care giver.
- The woman and her baby have a safe labor and birth.

PLACENTA PREVIA

Overview

In placenta previa the placenta is implanted in the lower uterine segment instead of the upper portion of the uterus. As the lower uterine segment contracts and dilates in the later weeks of pregnancy, the villi are torn from the uterine wall and bleeding results. If the placenta previa is complete, the placenta totally covers the internal cervical os. In partial placenta previa, a portion of the os is covered. Maternal risks are related to the possibility of hemorrhage and to psychologic stress resulting from concern about fetal well-being. Fetal-neonatal risks are related to the extent of the placenta previa. If a severe bleeding episode occurs the fetus often suffers fetal distress. Fetal demise is also a possibility if the condition is not diagnosed in a timely manner.

Medical Management

1. **Diagnosis.** Diagnosis is made based on a history of painless, bright red vaginal bleeding, especially in the third trimester. The initial bleeding episode may be light but is often followed by more severe bleeding. Diagnosis is confirmed with ultrasound to localize the placenta.

2. **Expectant management.** If < 37 weeks' gestation, expectant management is used to delay birth to allow the fetus to mature. This includes bed rest, no rectal or vaginal exams, monitoring of bleeding, ongoing assessment of fetal status with external monitor, monitoring of vital signs, laboratory evaluation (hemoglobin, hematocrit, Rh factor, urinalysis). Two units of cross-matched blood are kept available for transfusion. If the previa is partial or if the placenta is simply low-lying, vaginal birth may be attempted.

3. **Emergency management.** If severe bleeding occurs or evidence of fetal distress develops, a cesarean is performed.

Critical Nursing Assessments

1. Assess woman regularly for evidence of vaginal bleeding. If bleeding present, note amount, character.

2. Assess for signs of shock if bleeding present (decreased blood pressure, increased pulse, cool clammy skin, pallor, decreased hematocrit, urine output < 30 mL/hr).

3. Assess for uterine contractility and signs of labor. **Word of caution:** Vaginal exams may trigger a major bleeding episode and are **contraindicated.**

4. Assess woman's understanding of her condition, its implications, and treatment options.

5. Assess fetal status: During bleeding episode, continuous electronic fetal monitoring is used; when no bleeding is present, an electronic fetal monitoring strip is run, usually q4h (timing may vary according to agency policy).

Sample Nursing Diagnosis

- Altered tissue perfusion (placental) related to blood loss.
- Fear related to concern for own personal well-being and that of baby.

Critical Nursing Interventions

1. Carry out ongoing monitoring of maternal and fetal status including VS, evidence of bleeding, urinary output, electronic monitor tracing, signs of labor.

2. Explain procedures to woman and her family.

3. Administer IV fluids or blood products as ordered.

4. Review the following critical aspects of care you have provided:

   - Have I questioned the woman about bleeding? If bleeding is present, have I assessed quantity carefully?
   - Have I carefully monitored fetal status? Any signs of tachycardia? Decelerations?
   - Have I been alert for any changes in the woman's status? Any signs of labor? Any changes she has noted?
   - Have I implemented measures to help the woman be comfortable on bed rest—back rubs, positioning with pillows, diversionary activities?

Evaluation

- The woman's condition remains stable or, if bleeding occurs, it is detected promptly and therapy is begun.
- The woman and her baby have a safe labor and birth.

ADDITIONAL COMPLICATIONS

Table 2–1 describes additional complications that the nurse may encounter.

Table 2–1 Selected Complications During Pregnancy

Acquired Immunodeficiency Syndrome (AIDS)

Condition/Overview	Signs/Symptoms/Risk	Medical Therapy	Nursing Interventions
AIDS, caused by the human immunodeficiency virus, is a multisystem disorder that enters the body through blood, blood products, and bodily fluids such as semen, vaginal fluid, and urine. HIV affects T cells, thereby depressing the body's immune response. Persons at highest risk are homosexual or bisexual men, heterosexual partners of persons with AIDS, IV drug users, hemophiliacs, and fetuses of women at risk or HIV positive. Persons generally test positive for HIV within 6–12 weeks of exposure but may	The following women are considered at risk for AIDS: prostitutes; women with a history of sexually transmitted infection; IV drug users; partners (currently or previously) of IV drug users, bisexual men, hemophiliacs, or those who test positive for HIV. Women with AIDS may have any of the following: malaise, weight loss, lymphadenopathy, diarrhea, fever, neurologic dysfunction, immunodeficiency, esophageal candidiasis, herpes simplex virus, vaginal *Candida* infections, and cervical	Currently there is no definitive therapy for AIDS although a variety of experimental drugs are being tested. Current goal is to detect women at risk and educate the public about the spread of AIDS. Women at risk who are pregnant or planning a pregnancy should be offered HIV antibody testing. Women who test positive should be counseled about the implications for themselves and the fetus/newborn. They may be offered a therapeutic abortion. Women who continue pregnancy need	1. Assess history for risk factors. 2. Provide clear information about AIDS and the implications for the woman, her partner, and a child should the woman become pregnant. 3. Monitor asymptomatic pregnant woman for nonspecific symptoms such as fever, weight loss, persistent candidiasis (vaginal yeast infection or thrush in mouth), diarrhea, cough, skin lesions. 4. Implement appropriate isolation procedures

remain asymptomatic for five to ten years or more. In the U.S. the vast majority of pediatric AIDS cases have resulted from perinatal transmission from mother to child.

disease. Maternal risks: Progression of symptoms in HIV-positive, asymptomatic women may be accelerated by pregnancy.
Fetal–neonatal risks: Risk of transmission from HIV-positive mother to fetus. Infant often asymptomatic at birth; onset of symptoms usually occurs between 9 and 18 months. Facial characteristics that may indicate the newborn has been infected early in utero with HIV include microcephaly; patulous lips; prominent, boxlike forehead; increased distance between inner canthus of eyes; flattened nasal bridge.

excellent prenatal care with attention to psychosocial and teaching needs.

including use of disposable latex gloves when in contact with nonintact skin, mucous membranes, or bodily fluids (eg, changing chux, diapers, peripads, starting IV, drawing blood); use of protective covering such as plastic apron and glasses or eye shield when contamination from splashing may occur (vaginal exam, vaginal or cesarean birth, suctioning, care of newborn before initial bath). (Consult unit procedure manual for further specifics.)
5. Provide emotional support and nonjudgmental attitude; preserve confidentiality.

Continued

Table 2-1 continued

Condition/Overview	Signs/Symptoms/Risk	Medical Therapy	Nursing Interventions
Chlamydia			
Sexually transmitted infection caused by *Chlamydia trachomatis*, often found in association with gonorrhea.	Women are often asymptomatic. Symptoms may include thin or purulent vaginal discharge, frequency and burning with urination, or lower abdominal pain. Infant of woman with untreated chlamydia is at risk for newborn conjunctivitis, chlamydial pneumonia, preterm birth, or fetal demise.	Nonpregnant women treated with tetracycline. Because this may permanently discolor fetal teeth, pregnant women are treated with erythromycin ethyl succinate. Erythromycin ethyl ointment (but not silver nitrate) can prevent conjunctivitis in the newborn.	1. Review signs and symptoms, explain importance of taking entire dose of medication.
Gonorrhea			
Sexually transmitted infection caused by Neisseria gonorrhoeae.	Majority of women are asymptomatic; disease often diagnosed during routine prenatal cervical culture.	Pregnant women are treated with ceftriaxone plus erythromycin (CDC 1993). If the woman is allergic to	1. Review medication purpose, side effects. 2. Explain that untreated gonorrhea may result in

	If symptoms are present, they may include purulent vaginal discharge, dysuria, urinary frequency, inflammation and swelling of vulva. Cervix may appear eroded. Infection at time of birth may cause ophthalmia neonatorum in the newborn.	ceftriaxone, spectinomycin is used. All sexual partners are treated.	pelvic inflammatory disease and infertility. 3. Discuss safe sexual practices.
Syphilis Sexually transmitted infection caused by the spirochete *Treponema pallidum*.	Primary stage: chancre, slight fever, malaise. Chancre lasts about four weeks, then disappears. Secondary stage: occurs six weeks to six months after infection. Skin eruptions (condyloma lata); also symptoms of acute arthritis, liver enlargement, iritis, chronic sore throat with hoarseness.	For syphilis less than one year in duration: 2.4 million U benzathine penicillin G IM. For syphilis of more than one year's duration: 2.4 million U benzathine penicillin G once a week for three weeks. Sexual partners should also be screened and treated.	1. Explain the risk factors and long-term effects if syphilis is not treated. 2. Explain implications for fetus/neonate. 3. Stress importance of receiving all three doses if syphilis is greater than one year in duration.

Continued

Table 2–1   continued

Condition/Overview	Signs/Symptoms/Risk	Medical Therapy	Nursing Interventions
	Diagnosed by blood tests such as VDRL, RPR, FTA-ABS. Darkfield exam for spirochetes may be done. May be passed transplacentally to fetus. If untreated, one of the following can occur: second trimester abortion, stillborn infant at term, congenitally infected infant, uninfected live infant.		**Toxoplasmosis:** Explain methods of prevention to childbearing woman. She should avoid poorly cooked or raw meat, especially pork, beef, and lamb. Fruits and vegetables should be

TORCH

The TORCH group of infectious diseases may cause serious harm to fetus. They include toxoplasmosis (TO), rubella (R), cytomegalic inclusion disease (C), and herpes genitalis (H). Some	**Toxoplasmosis** results in a mild infection in adults but is associated with an increased risk of spontaneous abortion, prematurity, stillbirth, neonatal death, and disorders including micro-	**Toxoplasmosis:** Goal is to identify women at risk. Diagnosis made using serologic testing, physical findings, and history. Treatment includes sulfadiazine, pyrimethamine, and spira-	

sources identify the "O" as "other infections." Exposure of the woman during the first 12 weeks of pregnancy may cause developmental anomalies.

Toxoplasmosis is caused by a protozoan and transmitted by eating raw or poorly cooked meat or by exposure to feces of infected cats. Innocuous in adults.

Rubella or German measles is caused by a virus.

Cytomegalic inclusion disease (CID), caused by the cytomegalovirus (CMV), is the most prevalent infection of the TORCH group. Chronic persistent infection with viral shedding for years. Usually is asymptomatic in adults and children.

cephaly, hydrocephalus, convulsions, blindness, deafness, and mental retardation.

Rubella exposure in the first trimester is associated with spontaneous abortion, congenital heart disease, intrauterine growth retardation, cataracts, mental retardation, and cerebral palsy. Infection in the second trimester is most often associated with permanent hearing impairment in the newborn.

CID may cause fetal death; in neonates it is associated with microcephaly, cerebral palsy, mental retardation, etc. Subclinical infections may cause neurologic and hearing problems that may go unrecognized for months or years.

mycin. If toxoplasmosis is diagnosed before 20 weeks' gestation, therapeutic abortion may be offered because damage to the fetus tends to be more severe than if the disease is diagnosed later in pregnancy.

Rubella: Best therapy is prevention by vaccination. Women of childbearing age should be tested for immunity and vaccinated if susceptible. HAI titer of 1:16 or greater indicates immunity. Pregnant women are not vaccinated but will be offered vaccination postpartum. If infection occurs in first trimester, woman will be offered a therapeutic abortion.

CID: Diagnosis is confirmed by serologic tests to detect

washed. Litter box should be cleaned frequently by someone else, and woman should wear gloves when gardening.

Rubella: Assess for signs of rubella infection (maculopapular rash, lymphadenopathy, muscular achiness, joint pain). Provide emotional support and objective information for couples contemplating therapeutic abortion.

CID: Provide emotional support and objective information.

Herpes genitalis: Provide information about the disease and its spread. Advise woman to inform future health care providers of her infection. A possible association exists between herpes

Continued

Table 2–1 continued

Condition/Overview	Signs/Symptoms/Risk	Medical Therapy	Nursing Interventions
Herpes genitalis, caused by herpes simplex virus type 2 (HSV-2), is a chronic, recurring infection that causes painful lesions in the genital area and is transmitted by sexual contact.	**Herpes genitalis** may cause spontaneous abortion if active HSV-2 infection occurs in first trimester. Highest risk of infection for newborn who is born vaginally when mother has active HSV-2 in her vagina. Risk of neonatal death, permanent brain damage, characteristic skin lesions.	**CMV** antibodies. No effective treatment is available at this time. **Herpes genitalis:** Treatment is aimed at relieving woman's pain and may include sitz baths QID, followed by drying with a hair dryer; oral acyclovir reduces healing time but is not recommended during pregnancy. Oral acyclovir (Zovirax) does not cure infection or prevent recurrence but *does* reduce healing time. *Not* recommended for use in pregnancy. A cesarean birth is recommended for pregnant women with visible HSV-2 lesions; if no	and cervical cancer. Thus women should understand importance of yearly Pap smears. Provide emotional support and nonjudgmental attitude.

lesions are visible, vaginal birth is attempted. Vaginal birth is planned if membranes have been ruptured > 12 hours. Routine cultures during late pregnancy are no longer recommended but weekly examinations to detect the presence of lesions are recommended.

Substance Abuse

Indiscriminate use of alcohol or drugs such as cocaine, PCP, opiates, and methadone may affect the woman and her fetus/neonate. Alcohol abuse has been associated with fetal alcohol syndrome. Use of addicting drugs may cause the infant to be born addicted or to have serious and permanent problems.

Signs of addiction in the pregnant woman may include dilated or constricted pupils, inflamed nasal mucosa, abscesses, edema or track marks on arms and legs, inappropriate or disoriented behavior, or excessive fatigue.
Risks to the fetus include the following (varies somewhat according to substance

Following diagnosis, management involves a team approach to provide care for woman and fetus/neonate. Hospitalization may be necessary to achieve detoxification. "Cold turkey" withdrawal is not advised because of risk to fetus. Urine screening may be done regularly throughout the pregnancy

1. Be alert for signs of substance abuse. If it is suspected, ask direct questions, beginning with less threatening questions about use of tobacco, caffeine, and alcohol consumption. Then progress to questions about illicit drugs.
2. Provide information about the possible effects

Continued

Table 2–1 continued

Condition/Overview	Signs/Symptoms/Risk	Medical Therapy	Nursing Interventions
	abused): neurologic changes including marked irritability, poor interactive behavior, poor consolability, seizures, and so forth.	for women who are known or suspected substance abusers.	of substance abuse on the fetus.
Multiple Gestation			
Morbidity and mortality rates increase significantly in pregnancies with multiple fetuses. Dizygotic, or fraternal twins (resulting from two ova), are more common. Incidence of fraternal twins is affected by heredity, race, maternal age and parity, and fertility drugs. Monozygotic or identical twins (resulting from	Fetal risk is significantly higher. The perinatal mortality rate is higher, and there is an increased risk of preterm labor with the problems associated with prematurity. Multiple gestation increases the incidence of intrauterine growth retardation, congenital anomalies, and abnormal presentations. For the	Early diagnosis based on history, greater than anticipated uterine size. Ultrasound is crucial. Women are seen every two weeks until 28 weeks' gestation and then weekly. Serial ultrasounds are done regularly to assess for IUGR. NST and fetal biophysical profile are done at least weekly beginning at 28–30 weeks. Bed	1. Counsel on importance of good nutrition including adequate calories (40–45 kcal/kg/day), calcium (1800–2000 mg/day), and protein (more than 1.5 g/kg) (Garcia and Gall 1990). 2. Discuss importance of sufficient rest if at home (usually bed rest with BRP) or at least two

hours in the morning, afternoon, and evening.

3. If woman is hospitalized, explain importance of complete bed rest (or bed rest with BRP if ordered).

4. Monitor fetal status. This involves isolating each FHR as well as running an electronic fetal monitor strip on each fetus at least q4–8h (depending on agency policy). If possible the strips will be run at the same time using two (or three) monitors. This becomes more difficult with quadruplets.

5. Monitor for signs of complications such as PIH or preterm labor.

rest in the lateral position may be suggested as early as 23–26 weeks to prevent preterm labor. Maternal blood pressure is monitored closely. Preterm labor is managed in the same way as it is for single pregnancy (see earlier discussion in this chapter).

mother, a multiple gestation may contribute to more physical discomfort during pregnancy, such as shortness of breath, backaches, and pedal edema, as well as an increased incidence of PIH, anemia, and placenta previa. Prolonged hospitalization may be necessary, especially with three or more fetuses.

one ovum) are not as common. Incidence is not influenced by external factors other than infertility therapy. Higher numbers of fetuses (triplets or quadruplets, for example) may result from either process or a combination (Cunningham et al 1993).

REFERENCES

Centers for Disease Control and Prevention: 1993 Sexually transmitted disease treatment guidelines. *MMWR* 1993; 42(RR-14):4.

Cunningham FG et al: *Williams' Obstetrics,* 19th ed. Norwalk CT: Appleton & Lange, 1993.

Garcia PM, Gall SA: Multiple pregnancy. In: *Danforth's Obstetrics and Gynecology,* 6th ed. Scott JR et al (editors). Philadelphia: Lippincott, 1990.

Landon MB, Gable SG: Fetal surveillance in the pregnancy complicated by diabetes mellitus. *Clin Obstet Gynecol* 1991;34:535.

Mandeville L, Troiano N: *High-Risk Intrapartum Nursing.* Philadelphia: Lippincott, 1992.

Parsons MT, Spellacy WN: Causes and management of preterm labor. In: *Danforth's Obstetrics and Gynecology,* 7th ed. Scott JR et al (editors). Philadelphia: Lippincott, 1994.

Ratner R: Gestational diabetes mellitus: After three international workshops, do we know how to diagnose and manage it yet? *J Clin Endocrin Metabol* 1993; 77(1):1.

CHAPTER 3

The Intrapartal Client

OVERVIEW

Labor and birth progresses through four stages. A first time laboring woman (nullipara) will **average** twelve hours (11 hours in first stage and one hour of pushing in second stage). A multipara **averages** about eight hours (7-1/4 hours in first stage and 1/2 hour pushing in second stage). See Table 3–1 for definitions of each stage of labor and Table 3–2 for contraction and labor progress characteristics.

NURSING CARE DURING ADMISSION

Critical Nursing Assessments

Name: _____ Age: _____
   Maternal vital signs:
   BP_____ T_____ Radial pulse _____ R _____
   Gravida _____ Para _____ Term _____
   Preterm _____ Ab _____ Living _____
   EDB _____ Weeks gestation now _____
   Risk factors present _____
   Medications being taken _____
   Allergies: Medications _____ Foods _____
   Substances _____

Labor status

1. **Uterine contractions.** Ask mother and support person what the contraction pattern has been prior to admission. Assess uterine contractions by palpation on admission. Information regarding uterine

Table 3–1	Stages of Labor and Birth	
Stage	**Begins**	**Ends**
First	Beginning of cervical dilatation	Complete dilatation
Second	Complete dilatation	Birth of the baby
Third	Birth of the baby	Birth of the placenta
Fourth	Birth of the placenta	1–4 hours past birth

Table 3–2	Contraction and Labor Progress Characteristics

Contraction Characteristics

Latent phase:	Every 10–20 min × 15–20 seconds; mild, progressing to Every 5–7 min × 30–40 seconds; moderate
Active phase:	Every 2–3 min × 60 seconds; moderate to strong
Transition phase:	Every 2 min × 60–90 seconds; strong

Labor Progress Characteristics

Primipara:	1.2 cm/hr dilatation 1 cm/hr descent < 2 hr in second stage
Multipara:	1.5 cm/hr dilatation 2 cm/hr descent < 1 hr in second stage

contractions will be needed to determine labor status, fetal status, and the need for further nursing interventions.

Assessment Technique: With the woman's gown over her abdomen, but blankets pulled aside, place palmar surface of fingers on fundus of uterus (upper portion, above the umbilicus). During your assessment and evaluation you will determine contraction frequency, duration, and intensity. When uterine tightening begins, note the time (use second hand on a clock or watch), continue to assess the tighten-

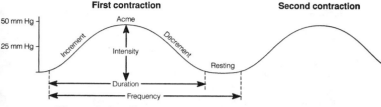

Figure 3–1   Characteristics of uterine contractions.

ing, and when it has completely relaxed, once again note the time. (This provides information regarding duration of that contraction.) Continue to watch the time and note the beginning of the next contraction. This will establish frequency (from the beginning of one contraction to the beginning of the next contraction.) (See Figure 3–1.) While feeling the tightening, slightly push your fingertips against the uterus. If the tissue indents easily, the intensity is mild; if it indents a small amount, the intensity is moderate; if it indents a very small amount, the intensity is strong. Contraction frequency and duration may also be assessed and evaluated by using external electronic monitoring. Contraction intensity may be measured more precisely by use of an intrauterine uterine pressure device that attaches to the electronic monitor.

2. **Cervical dilatation and effacement.** Cervical dilatation progresses from 0 to 10 cm and effacement progresses from 0% to 100%.
   Assessment technique: See Procedure 15: Sterile Vaginal Exam, and Figure 3–2.

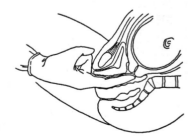

Figure 3–2   Determination of cervical dilatation.

3. **Amniotic fluid membrane status.** Amniotic membranes are either intact or ruptured. If ruptured, the time of rupture needs to be noted and the fluid is observed for amount (usually described as small, moderate, or large) (remember, there is about 600–800 mL of fluid at 40 weeks' gestation), color (should be colorless), odor (should be nonfoul), and consistency (should be clear; cloudy fluid may indicate infection, and meconium may be associated with fetal stress).
   Assessment technique: See Procedure 15: Sterile Vaginal Exam and Procedure 2: Assessment for Amniotic Fluid.

Essential Precautions in Practice

During Intrapartal Assessment

Examples of times when disposable gloves should be worn include the following:

- Assisting the woman as she removes any garments moist with bloody show and/or amniotic fluid
- Handling chux and bedding that are moist with bloody show and/or amniotic fluid
- Checking amniotic fluid-soaked materials with Nitrazine test tape
- Placing the elastic straps for the electronic monitor around a woman who has been lying in bedding moist with bloody show and/or amniotic fluid
- Assisting with fetal blood sampling and handling the lab tubes

Wear sterile gloves when performing a sterile vaginal exam and placing fetal scalp electrodes. The sterile gloves are used to maintain sterile asepsis. They protect the nurse from exposure to vaginal secretions, bloody show, and amniotic fluid.

REMEMBER to wash your hands prior to pulling the disposable gloves on and AGAIN immediately after you remove the gloves.

For further information consult OSHA and CDC guidelines.

4. **Fetal status.**
   a. **Fetal heart rate (FHR).** When auscultating the FHR, the nurse determines rate, regularity, and whether slowing is heard during or just after uterine contractions. Assess FHR with the woman in high Fowler's (back of the bed is almost completely upright), in semi-Fowler's (back of bed is at approximately 45 degrees), or in side-lying position (to maximize blood flow to the fetus). When assessing the FHR by electronic fetal monitor (EFM), the nurse gathers data regarding baseline fetal heart rate, variability (short-term and long-term), and periodic changes (accelerations and decelerations). Once these data are known, the nurse can evaluate the tracing as reassuring (a normal pattern), or nonreassuring (a pattern that may be associated with fetal distress of some type).
   Assessment technique—auscultation: The FHR may be auscultated with a fetoscope or a hand-held ultrasound device. See Procedure 6: Fetal Heart Rate Auscultation.
   Assessment technique—electronic fetal monitoring: See Procedure 7: Fetal Monitoring: Electronic. A sample of a tracing is illustrated in Figure 3–3. Note that time is assessed by counting the squares or the darker vertical lines.
   Terms related to fetal heart rate monitoring include the following:
   Baseline rate: Refers to the range of FHR observed between contractions during a ten-minute period of monitoring. The range does not include the rate present during decelerations.
   Baseline changes: Defined in terms of ten-minute periods of time. Changes include: tachycardia, bradycardia, and variability of heart rate.
   Tachycardia: FHR 160 beats per minute (bpm) or more for more than ten minutes; moderate (160–179 bpm), severe (180 or more).
   Bradycardia: FHR less than 120 bpm for more than ten minutes; mild (100–119 bpm), moderate (less than 100 bpm), severe (less than 70 bpm). Other characteristics of EFM tracings are presented in Table 3–3.

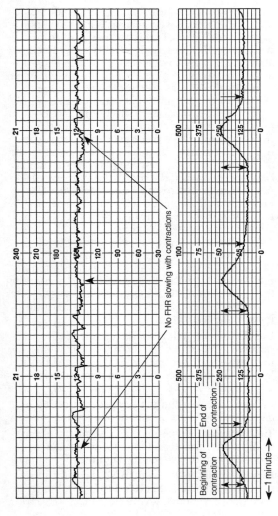

Figure 3-3   Normal FHR range is from 120 to 160 bpm. The FHR tracing in the upper portion of the graph indicates FHR range of 140–155 bpm. The lower portion is a tracing of the uterine contraction pattern (frequency and duration of contractions).

Table 3–3 Characteristics of FHR Tracings

Example	Characteristic	Nursing Intervention
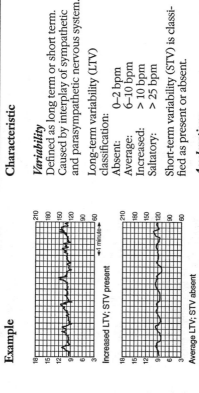 Increased LTV; STV present Average LTV; STV absent Absent LTV; STV present	*Variability* Defined as long term or short term. Caused by interplay of sympathetic and parasympathetic nervous system. Long-term variability (LTV) classification: Absent: 0–2 bpm Average: 6–10 bpm Increased: > 10 bpm Saltatory: > 25 bpm Short-term variability (STV) is classified as present or absent. *Accelerations* An increase of FHR that lasts for a few seconds Occurs with fetal movement Is basis of nonstress test (NST).	Maximize uteroplacental perfusion by positioning woman on left side. Document findings. Report status to certified nurse-midwife (CNM) or physician. Correct maternal hypotension by turning woman to side-lying position, increasing rate of intravenous infusion. For the most part, there are no specific interventions. 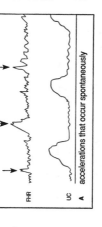 FHR UC ▲ accelerations that occur spontaneously

Example	Characteristic	Nursing Intervention
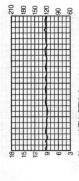 Absent LTV; STV absent	**Deceleration** Periodic decreases in FHR from the normal baseline. Classified as early, late, or variable.	No specific intervention needed. Monitor for changes in FHR pattern.
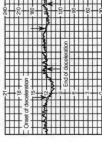 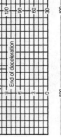 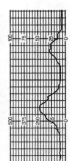	**Early deceleration** Due to pressure on the fetal head as it progresses down the birth canal. Characteristics: Resembles upside down shape of uterine contraction. Occurs at or just before the beginning of contraction and ends as contraction ends. Nadir (lowest point) occurs at peak of contraction, and is within normal FHR range. Is considered a normal variation.	Evaluate for possible cephalopelvic disproportion (CPD) if occurs in early labor.

Table 3–3 continued

Late deceleration

Due to uteroplacental insufficiency as the result of decreased blood flow and oxygen transfer to the fetus during contractions.

Characteristics:
Smooth, uniform shape that inversely mirrors contraction.

Begin at or within seconds after the peak of the contraction.

Last past end of contraction.

Tend to occur with every contraction; they are persistent and consistent.

Usually occur within normal FHR range.

In some situations, changing maternal position, providing IV hydration, and decreasing contraction frequency decrease late decelerations.

Turn woman to left side-lying position.

Report findings to physician/CNM and document findings.

Provide explanation to woman and partner.

Monitor for further FHR changes.

Maintain good hydration with IV fluids.

Discontinue oxytocin if it is being administered.

Administer oxygen by face mask at 7–10 L/min.

Monitor maternal BP, P for signs of hypotension.

Assist with preparation for cesarean birth if required.

Variable deceleration

Due to umbilical cord compression, which decreases the amount of blood flow (therefore oxygen supply) to the fetus.

Document findings.

Report status to certified nurse-midwife/physician.

Continued

Table 3–3	continued	
Example	**Characteristic**	**Nursing Intervention**
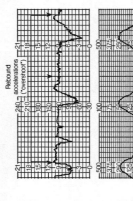	Characteristics: Vary in onset, occurrence, and waveform.	Change maternal position to one in which FHR pattern is most improved.
		Correct maternal hypotension.
	Usually fall outside the normal FHR range.	Assist with preparation for cesarean birth if required.
	Are acute in onset.	Provide explanation to woman and partner.
		Discontinue oxytocin if it is being administered and there are severe variables. Oxytocin may be continued if mild or moderate decelerations are present.
		Perform vaginal examination to assess for prolapsed cord or change in labor progress.
		Monitor FHR continuously to assess current status and for further changes in FHR pattern.

b. **Evaluation of fetal heart rate tracings.**
Although it seems an awkward way to begin, evaluation of the electronic monitor tracing begins by looking at the uterine contraction pattern. To evaluate the contraction pattern the nurse should:
   1. Determine the uterine resting tone.
   2. Assess the contractions:
      What is the frequency?
      What is the duration?
      What is the intensity (if internal monitoring)?

   The next step is to evaluate the fetal heart rate tracing.

   1. Determine the baseline:
      Is the baseline within normal range?
      Is there evidence of tachycardia?
      Is there evidence of bradycardia?
   2. Determine FHR variability:
      Is short-term variability present or absent?
      Is long-term variability average? Minimal to absent?
      Moderate to marked?
   3. Is a sinusoidal pattern present?
   4. Are there periodic changes?
      Are accelerations present?
      Do they meet the criteria for a reactive non-stress test (NST)?
      Are decelerations present?
      Are they uniform in shape? If so, determine if they are early or late decelerations.
      Are they nonuniform in shape? If so, determine if they are variable decelerations.

c. **Classifying the FHR tracing as reassuring or nonreassuring.** After evaluating the FHR tracing for the factors just listed, the nurse may further classify the tracing as reassuring or nonreassuring. A reassuring pattern is as follows: FHR between 120–160 bpm, STV present, LTV average, accelerations with fetal movement, absence of late or variable deceleration. If the pattern is reassuring, no additional treatment or intervention is required. If the pattern is nonreassuring, continuous monitoring and more involved treatment and intervention may be required.

5. **Fetal presentation and position.** Fetal position refers to the relationship of the fetal presenting part (the part of the fetus that enters the maternal pelvis first) to the maternal pelvis, for example: right occiput anterior (ROA) or left occiput anterior (LOA). Fetal presentation may be cephalic, breech, or transverse. Cephalic presentation is the most common and occurs in 97% of births. Breech presentation occurs just under 3% of the time.
   Assessment technique: Fetal presentation and position are determined by vaginal examination. See Procedure 15: Sterile Vaginal Exam and Figure 3–4.

6. **Information, comfort, coping level and available support.** Assessment of the woman's physical and emotional state, her coping methods and her support system will provide useful information for the admission process and later in the labor.
   Assessment technique: In a conversational interview format, determine the type of prenatal education program the woman has completed. What

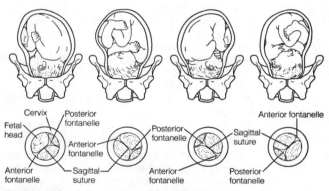

Figure 3–4 Assessment of fetal position. A, Left occiput anterior (LOA). The posterior fontanelle (triangle-shaped) is in the upper left quadrant of the maternal pelvis. B, Left occiput posterior (LOP). The posterior fontanelle is in the lower left quadrant of the maternal pelvis. C, Right occiput anterior (ROA). The posterior fontanelle is in the upper right quadrant of the maternal pelvis. D, Right occiput posterior (ROP). The posterior fontanelle is in the lower right quadrant of the maternal pelvis.

hopes and plans does she have for this birth? Has she completed a birth plan or made a formalized list of special requests during the labor and birth? What plans has she made with the certified nurse-midwife/physician? Does she verbalize the need for information or does she have questions? Does she have a resource/support person with her?

Assessment of psychosocial history is a critical component of intrapartal nursing assessment. The nurse begins the assessment when the woman is admitted into the birthing area by obtaining information such as the following:

a. What is her marital status? Who are her support people? Is there evidence of support between the woman and her partner? Is the partner controlling? Does the partner make decisions unilaterally? Does the partner speak for the woman and answer all the questions?

b. Is she safe in her relationship with the baby's father? Has there been any physical or emotional abuse prior to or during the pregnancy? If so, what interventions were made? In questioning the woman about safety and abuse issues it is important for the nurse to be aware that abuse affects one in six adult women and one in five teenagers during pregnancy (McFarland & Parker 1994). It is important to ensure that the woman is alone when the questions are asked so that she can answer freely. If she indicates there has been a problem, the questions from the Abuse Assessment Screen by McFarland and Parker (1994, p 322) could be used. The questions include:

   1. Have you ever been emotionally or physically abused by your partner or someone important to you?
   2. Within the last year, have you been hit, slapped, kicked, or otherwise physically hurt by someone? If yes, by whom? Total number of times?
   3. Since you've been pregnant, were you hit, slapped, kicked, or otherwise physically hurt by someone? If yes, by whom? Total number of times?

Table 3–4   Deviations from Normal Labor Process Requiring Immediate Intervention

Finding	Immediate Action	Finding	Immediate Action
Woman admitted with unusual vaginal bleeding or history of painless vaginal bleeding	1. Do not perform vaginal examination. 2. Assess FHR. 3. Evaluate amount of blood loss. 4. Evaluate labor pattern. 5. Notify physician/CNM immediately.	Prolapse of umbilical cord	1. Relieve pressure on cord manually. 2. Continuously monitor FHR; watch for changes in FHR pattern. 3. Notify physician/CNM. 4. Assist woman into knee-chest position. 5. Administer oxygen. 6. Direct another person to prepare for immediate cesarean section. 7. Watch for decreasing baseline, loss of variability, presence of late or variable decelerations.
Presence of greenish or brownish amniotic fluid	1. Continuously monitor FHR. 2. Evaluate dilatation status of cervix and determine whether umbilical cord is prolapsed. 3. Evaluate presentation (vertex or breech). 4. Maintain woman on complete bed rest on left side. 5. Notify physician/CNM immediately. 6. Note color and consistency of amniotic fluid.		

Absence of FHR and fetal movement

1. Notify physician/CNM.
2. Provide truthful information and emotional support to laboring couple.
3. Remain with the couple.
4. Prepare for diagnostic ultrasound exam.

Woman admitted in advanced labor; birth imminent

1. Prepare for immediate birth.
2. Obtain critical information:
   a. EDB
   b. History of bleeding problems
   c. History of medical or obstetrical problems
   d. Past and or present use/abuse of prescription/OTC/illicit drugs
   e. Problems with this pregnancy
   f. FHR and maternal vital signs if possible
   g. Whether membranes are ruptured and how long since rupture
   h. Blood type and Rh
3. Direct another person to contact CNM/physician. Do not leave woman alone.
4. Provide support to couple.
5. Put on gloves.

4. Within the last year has anyone forced you to have sexual activities? If yes, who? Total number of times?
5. Are you afraid of your partner or anyone you listed above?

It is important for the nurse to obtain the history in a setting that promotes trust and the establishment of a relationship. Some of the questions are straightforward, but others require care and privacy to ensure that the woman has a safe environment in which to address them.

7. **Assessment findings that require immediate intervention.** See Table 3–4.

Sample admission nursing note   Grav I Para 0 EDB 1-13-96 40 wks gest admitted ambulatory to BR1 in labor. Contractions q3 X 50 of mod qual. Memb intact. Cervix 5 cm, 80% effaced, soft and anterior, Bishop score 12. Small amount blood-tinged mucus present. Vertex presentation at 0 station. FHR 140 by auscultation, regular rhythm. No increase or decrease in FHR noted during or following UC. Maternal temp 98.6, pulse 78, resp 18, BP 120/74. Adm UA obtained and to lab. Support person with pt and to remain through birth. P. Gomez, RNC

NURSING CARE DURING LABOR

Critical Nursing Assessments

Additional assessments of maternal and fetal status and labor progress are presented in Table 3–5.

Critical Nursing Interventions

1. During labor, the nursing support measures will vary depending on the progress of labor and the wishes of the laboring woman or couple. Table 3–6 summarizes the major characteristics of labor and birth and presents nursing interventions that may be used in each stage of labor.

2. Teach a visualization method. If the woman is in early labor or is awaiting an induction, there is time

Table 3–5 Nursing Assessments During Labor and Birth

Stage	Maternal Assessments	Fetal Assessments
First Stage Latent phase	Blood pressure, pulse, respirations q1hr if in normal range. Temperature q4hr unless over 37.5C (99.6F) or membranes ruptured, then q1hr. Uterine contractions q30min.	FHR q60min for low-risk women and q30min for high-risk women, if normal characteristics present (average variability, baseline in the 120–160 bpm range, without late or variable decelerations [NAACOG 1990]). Note fetal activity. If EFM in place, assess for reactive NST.
Active phase	BP, P, R q1hr if in normal range. Uterine contractions q30min.	FHR q30min for low-risk women and q15min for high-risk women, if normal characteristics are present (NAACOG 1990).
Transition	BP, P, R q30min.	FHR q30min for low-risk women and every 15 min for high-risk women.
Second Stage	BP, P, R q5–15min. Uterine contractions palpated with each contraction or continuously.	FHR q15min for low-risk women and q5min for high-risk women (NAACOG 1990).

NAACOG 1990.

Table 3–6   Normal Progress, Psychologic Characteristics, and Nursing Support During First and Second Stages of Labor

Stage / Phase	Cervical Dilatation	Uterine Contractions	Woman's Response	Nursing Support Measures
Stage 1 Latent phase:	1–4 cm	Every 15–30 min, 15–30 sec duration. Mild intensity	Usually happy, talkative, and eager to be in labor. Exhibits need for independence by taking care of own bodily needs and seeking information	Establish rapport on admission and continue to build during care. Assess information base and learning needs. Be available to consult regarding breathing technique if needed; teach breathing technique if needed and in early labor. Orient family to room, equipment, monitors, and procedures. Encourage woman and partner to participate in care as desired. Provide needed information. Assist woman into position of comfort (nonsupine position); encourage frequent change of position; and encourage ambulation during early labor. Offer fluids/ice chips. Keep couple informed of progress. Encourage woman to void every one to two hours. Assess need for and interest in using visualization to enhance relaxation and teach if appropriate.

Active phase:	4–7 cm	Every 3–5 min, 30–60 sec duration Moderate intensity	May experience feelings of helplessness; exhibits increased fatigue and may begin to feel restless and anxious as contractions become stronger; expresses fear of abandonment Becomes more dependent as she is less able to meet her needs	Observe response to contractions. Encourage woman to maintain breathing patterns; provide quiet environment to reduce external stimuli. Provide reassurance, encouragement, support; keep couple informed of progress. Promote comfort by giving backrubs, sacral pressure, cool cloth on forehead, assistance with position changes, support with pillows, effleurage. Provide ice chips, ointment for dry mouth and lips. Encourage to void every one to two hours. Offer shower/Jacuzzi/warm bath if available.
Transition:	8–10 cm	Every 2–3 min, 45–90 sec duration Strong intensity	Tires and may exhibit increased restlessness and irritability; may feel she cannot keep up with labor process and is out of control Physical discomforts Fear of being left alone May fear tearing open or splitting apart with contractions	Encourage woman to rest between contractions; if she sleeps between contractions, wake her at beginning of contraction so she can begin breathing pattern (increases feeling of control). Provide support, encouragement, and praise for efforts. Keep couple informed of progress; encourage continued participation of support persons. Promote comfort as listed above but recognize many women do not want to be touched when in transition. Provide privacy. Provide ice chips, ointment

Continued

Table 3–6 continued

Stage / Phase	Cervical Dilatation	Uterine Contractions	Woman's Response	Nursing Support Measures
				for lips. Encourage to void every one to two hours. If she has difficulty focusing, cup your hands close to her face and place your face close to hers. Talk her through the contraction. Have her breathe with you.
Stage 2	Complete	Every 1-1/2 –2 minutes	May feel out of control, helpless, panicky, exhausted, exhilarated	Assist woman in pushing efforts. Encourage woman to assume position of comfort. She may be most comfortable in a sitting position on a toilet, leaning over a birthing bar, on hands and knees, or perhaps on her side. Some women like to sit in high Fowler's, to have support behind their shoulders, and to have someone hold their legs up and flexed while they push. Provide encouragement and praise for efforts. Keep couple informed of progress. Provide ice chips and cool cloth for forehead. Maintain privacy as woman desires.

to teach her a visualization technique that can be used during labor. Direct a visualization by saying something like the following: "Think about a place you have been that has pleasant memories and feelings around it. A place that was relaxing, where all your stress disappeared. As you think about this, take in a breath and remember the smells around the place. If it was outside, feel the warmth of the sun or the way the breeze felt on your face. In your mind, sit in that place again. Let all your tension and tiredness leave your body as you feel the warmth and breezes."

Give the woman a few moments to think about her special place. Ask if she would like to share information about the setting. If the woman chooses to do this add the information to help her with the visualization (for example, "think about the mountain cabin and the warmth of the sun on your face as you sit in the rocking chair on the front porch," etc).

After the woman has a visualization set up, suggest thinking about it during contractions as a means of increasing relaxation and focusing concentration. You could say: "As each contraction begins, think about this special place for a moment and let your body relax. Keep a picture of your place in your mind as you breathe with the contraction. When the contraction is over, let your body stay relaxed. Feel the comfort of this room and support of those around you."

3. Teach a progressive relaxation sequence. If the woman is just beginning labor, you may have an opportunity to teach a relaxation exercise. Instruct her as follows:

   a. Assume a comfortable position (mid-Fowler's with arms supported by pillows, or side-lying with pillow between knees and pillows to support arms, or in a reclining or rocking chair).
   b. Breathe slowly and easily. Close your eyes and let your body sink into the bed (or chair). Adjust your position so that each part of your body is supported and comfortable.
   c. Maintain your breathing and try to keep your mind clear. To help focus, think of the number 1 as you inhale, and the number 2 as you exhale.

Each time your mind begins to drift away, quietly think about the numbers.

d. Tighten your face, hold it a few seconds, and then release all the tightness. Let it flow out with your breath.
Note: After doing this exercise the first time, the woman may want to do the progressive relaxation exercise by herself, or may want her support person to talk through it with her.

e. Tighten, hold, and then release the neck and shoulders ... the right arm and hand ... the left arm and hand ... the chest and upper back ... the abdomen ... the right thigh ... the right lower leg, ankle, and foot ... the left thigh ... the left lower leg, ankle, and foot.
Note: A variation of this exercise is to have the woman tighten the body part, hold for a few seconds, and then release it as the coach lightly strokes that body part. Later in labor, gentle stroking of the woman's arms or back will enhance relaxation.

4. Teach paced breathing. Determine which breathing method the woman (couple) has learned. Provide encouragement as needed in maintaining breathing pattern. Provide support to the labor coach and assist as needed.

Lamaze breathing pattern cues

First-level breathing Pattern begins and ends with a cleansing breath (in through the nose and out through pursed lips as if cooling a spoonful of hot food). While inhaling through the nose and exhaling through pursed lips, slow breaths are taken moving only the chest. The rate should be approximately 6–9/minute or two breaths/15 seconds. The coach or nurse may assist by reminding the woman to take a cleansing breath and then the breaths could be counted out if needed to maintain pacing.

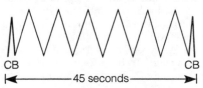

The woman inhales as someone counts "one one thousand, two one thousand, three one thousand, four one thousand." Exhalation begins and continues through the same count.

Second-level breathing Pattern begins and ends with a cleansing breath. Breaths are then taken in and out silently through the mouth at approximately four breaths/5 seconds. The jaw and entire body needs to be relaxed. The rate can be accelerated to 2–2-1/2 breaths/second. The rhythm for the breaths can be counted out as "one and two and one and two and ..." with the woman exhaling on the numbers and inhaling on *and.*

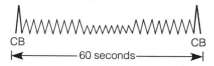

Third-level breathing Pattern begins and ends with a cleansing breath. All breaths are rhythmical, in and out through the mouth. Exhalations are accompanied by a "Hee" or "Hoo" sound in a varying pattern, which begins as 3:1 (Hee Hee Hee Hoo) and can change to 2:1 (Hee Hee Hoo) or 1:1 (Hee Hoo) as the intensity of the contraction changes. The rate should not be more rapid than 2–2-1/2/second. The rhythm of the breaths would match a "one and two and ..." count.

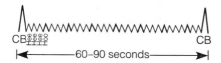

Abdominal breathing pattern cues

The abdomen moves outward during inhalation and downward during exhalation. The rate remains slow with approximately 6–9 breaths/minute.

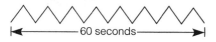

Quick method

When the woman has not learned a particular method and is in active phase of labor, the nurse may teach her a combination of two patterns. Abdominal breathing may be used until labor is more advanced. Then a more rapid pattern can be used consisting of two short blows from the mouth followed by a longer blow. (This pattern is called "pant pant blow" even though all exhalations are a blowing motion.)

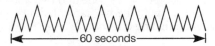

|←————— 60 seconds —————→|

5. Administer analgesic agents as needed. The guidelines for administration are as follows:

   - Assess woman and her record for history of allergies.

   - Assess baseline FHR and maternal vital signs prior to administration of analgesic in order to have a comparison if hypotension or FHR changes occur. Record findings on the chart and on EFM strip (if running).

   - Encourage woman to empty her bladder prior to administration of analgesic to enhance the rest and relaxation from the drug.

   - Raise side rails to provide safety and explain this precaution to client.

   - Monitor maternal vital signs and FHR to assure they remain in a normal range.

   - Chart analgesic administration and maternal-fetal status on client record and on EFM tracing.
     Note: Analgesics are not given if the maternal vital signs are unstable, if the woman is hypotensive, if severe hemorrhage is present, or if the baby is preterm.

6. Provide nursing support during regional blocks. See Table 3–7, which highlights nursing actions during regional blocks.

Table 3–7 Summary of Commonly Used Regional Blocks			
Type of Block	Area Affected	Use During Labor and Birth	Nursing Actions
Lumbar epidural	Vagina and perineum	Given in first stage and second stage of labor	Assess woman's knowledge regarding the block. Act as advocate to help her obtain further information if needed. Monitor maternal blood pressure to detect the major side effect, which is hypotension. Provide support and comfort.
Pudendal	Perineum and lower vagina	Given in the second stage just prior to birth to provide anesthesia for episiotomy or for low forceps delivery	Assess woman's knowledge regarding the block. Act as advocate to help her obtain further information if needed.
Local infiltration	Perineum	Administered just before birth to provide anesthesia for episiotomy	Assess woman's knowledge regarding the block. Provide information as needed. Provide comfort and support. Observe perineum for bruising or other discoloration in the recovery period.

NURSING CARE AT THE TIME OF BIRTH

Critical Nursing Assessments

1. Assessments are outlined in Table 3–5 on page 81.

Critical Nursing Interventions

1. Prepare the birthing area as the time of birth approaches.
2. The certified nurse-midwife/physician is summoned if not already present.
3. Maternal-fetal assessments are continued as outlined in Table 3–5.
4. The nurse and support person assist the woman in her pushing efforts.
5. An instrument table and other equipment are prepared.
6. Oxygen and suction equipment is readied if needed for both mother and newborn.
7. Identification bracelets are prepared.
8. Just prior to the birth, the nurse dons sterile gloves and cleanses the perineum.

NURSING CARE IMMEDIATELY AFTER THE BIRTH OF THE BABY

Critical Nursing Assessments

1. Assess the Apgar score for the newborn at one and five minutes of age (see Table 3–8).
2. Complete an initial physical assessment of the newborn (see Table 3–9).

Critical Nursing Interventions

1. Don disposable gloves when handling the newborn.
2. Provide warmth for the newborn by drying with warmed soft blankets, placing under a radiant warmer, or by placing the newborn skin to skin with the mother.

Table 3–8   The Apgar Scoring System*

Sign	Score		
	0	1	2
Heart rate	Absent	Slow—below 100	Above 100
Respiratory effort	Absent	Slow—irregular	Good crying
Muscle tone	Flaccid	Some flexion of extremities	Active motion
Reflex irritability	None	Grimace	Vigorous cry
Color	Pale blue	Body pink, blue extremities	Completely pink

*From Apgar V: The newborn (Apgar) scoring system: reflections and advice. *Pediatric Clin North Am* 1966; 13 (August): 645.

3. Maintain a clear airway in the newborn by suctioning with the bulb syringe or by using nasopharyngeal suctioning if needed (see Procedure 16: Suctioning of the Newborn).

4. Prevent infection in the newborn by washing hands thoroughly prior to the birth, maintaining asepsis in placing the umbilical cord clamp, and maintaining asepsis if eye prophylaxis is administered in the birthing area.

5. Ensure correct identification of the newborn by placing identification bracelets on the mother and newborn at birth (in some institutions, an identification band is also placed on the support person), and obtaining newborn's footprints and maternal finger print on birth record.

6. Continue to provide support to the woman and her partner.

7. Maintain birth record for the client chart.

8. Monitor maternal blood pressure (BP) and pulse (P).

9. Administer oxytocin as ordered by physician/certified nurse-midwife (see Drug Guide 7: Oxytocin

Table 3–9   Initial Newborn Evaluation

Assess	Normal Findings
Respirations	Rate 30–60 irregular No retractions, no grunting
Apical pulse	Rate 120–160 and somewhat irregular
Temperature	Skin temp above 97.8F (36.5C)
Skin color	Body pink with bluish extremities
Umbilical cord	Two arteries and one vein
Gestational age	Should be 38–42 weeks to remain with parents for extended time
Sole creases	Sole creases that involve the heel

In general expect: scant amount of vernix on upper back, axilla, groin; lanugo only on upper back; ears with incurving of upper 2/3 of pinnae and thin cartilage that springs back from folding; male genitalia—testes palpated in upper or lower scrotum; female genitalia—labia majora larger; clitoris nearly covered.

In the following situations, newborns should generally be stabilized rather than remaining with parents in the birth area for an extended period of time:

Apgar is less than 8 at one minute and less than 9 at five minutes, or a baby requires resuscitation measures (other than whiffs of oxygen).
Respirations are below 30 or above 60, with retractions and/or grunting.
Apical pulse is below 120 or above 160 with marked irregularities.
Skin temperature is below 97.8F (36.5C).
Skin color is pale blue, or there is circumoral pallor.
Baby is less than 38 or more than 42 weeks' gestation.
Baby is very small or very large for gestational age.
There are congenital anomalies involving open areas in the skin (meningomyelocele).

[Pitocin]). The oxytocin may be added to the IV solution if one has already been started, or may be given IM (frequently the ventrogluteal or vastas lateralis site is used).

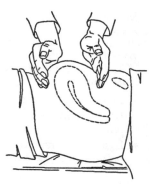

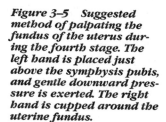

Figure 3–5 Suggested method of palpating the fundus of the uterus during the fourth stage. The left hand is placed just above the symphysis pubis, and gentle downward pressure is exerted. The right hand is cupped around the uterine fundus.

NURSING CARE IN THE IMMEDIATE RECOVERY PERIOD (FOURTH STAGE)

Critical Nursing Assessments

Complete maternal assessments q15 X 4, q30 X 2, q1–2hr X two. Maternal BP and pulse are obtained first, then the uterine fundus is assessed (see Figure 3–5). After removing the peripad or chux, the perineum is observed for

Table 3–10   Maternal Adaptations Following Birth

Characteristic	Normal Findings
Blood pressure	Should return to prelabor level
Pulse	Slightly lower than in labor
Uterine fundus	In the midline at the umbilicus or 1–2 fingerbreadths below the umbilicus
Lochia	Red (rubra), small to moderate amount (from spotting on pads to 1/4–1/2 of pad covered in 15 minutes). Should not exceed saturation of one pad in first hour
Bladder	Nonpalpable
Perineum	Smooth, pink, without bruising or edema
Emotional state	Wide variation, including excited, exhilarated smiling, crying, fatigue, verbal, quiet, pensive, and sleepy

swelling, bruising, or lacerations. The amount of lochia is also assessed (see Procedure 4: Evaluation of Lochia after Birth). During the assessment the nurse may anticipate the findings indicated in Table 3–10.

The frequent assessments of the immediate recovery cease when:

- Blood pressure and pulse are stable.
- Uterus is firm, in the midline, and below the umbilicus.
- Lochia is rubra, moderate in amount, without clots.
- Perineum is free from bruising or excessive edema.

Critical Nursing Interventions

Support parental attachment by providing private time for the parents and the newborn. Encourage the mother to hold the infant as she desires. Facilitate eye contact by turning down the lights in the recovery area. If this is the first baby, some parents enjoy looking the baby over with the nurse explaining some of the newborn characteristics. Monitor newborn status (temperature, skin color, respiratory and heart rate, and need for oral suctioning).

REFERENCES

McFarland J, Parker B: Preventing abuse during pregnancy: An assessment and intervention protocol. *Matern Child Nurs* 1994;19:321.

CHAPTER 4

The At-Risk Intrapartal Client

FAILURE TO PROGRESS IN LABOR

Overview

Failure to progress in labor is defined as no progress in cervical dilatation or descent of the presenting part during active labor. Failure to progress may be associated with malpresentation (breech, transverse, face or brow), malposition (occiput posterior), or cephalopelvic disproportion (CPD). When such conditions are recognized and treated aggressively, 50% of women will have vaginal birth, while the other 50% will require cesarean birth (Lipshitz 1990).

Maternal risks include infection secondary to increased number of vaginal examinations to determine status, dehydration secondary to inadequate fluid intake, and exhaustion associated with lengthening of the labor. Fetal risks include stress from maternal dehydration and subsequent hypotension and from prolonged labor.

Medical Management

1. **Fluid therapy.** Intravenous fluids may be ordered to rehydrate the laboring woman.

2. **Rule out CPD.** Clinical evaluation or x-ray pelvimetry may be used. Clinical evaluation (pelvimetry) involves the physician evaluating cervical dilatations, fetal descent (station), and fetal position. Then oxytocin is begun to ensure that adequate uterine contractions occur. After one hour of adequate uterine contractions, cervical dilatation and fetal station is reevaluated. If progress has been made, labor continues. If no progress has occurred, a cesarean

birth occurs. X-ray pelvimetry may be used as an alternate evaluation method.

3. **Stimulation of labor.** If CPD is ruled out (or clinical pelvimetry is done) and uterine contractions are less than normal in frequency and quality, an oxytocin infusion may be started to augment the labor pattern.

4. **Method of birth.** If CPD is present, cesarean birth is advised.

Critical Nursing Assessments

1. Maintain excellent clinical practice that protects you from body substances and fluids.

2. Assess fetal vertex for engagement into the maternal pelvis. If engaged, the fetal head is at the level of the ischial spines on vaginal examination.

3. Assess uterine contractions. Normal contractions occur every two to three minutes, lasting 50–60 seconds, and are of moderate to strong intensity. If when palpated contraction intensity is less than expected (for this point in labor) and the amount of pain the woman experiences seems out of proportion (feels pain before contraction begins, intense discomfort during contraction, and pain after the

---

Essential Precautions in Practice

During Care of the Woman at Risk for Intrapartal Complications

Examples of times when disposable gloves should be worn include:

- Handling chux and bedding that are moist with bloody show or amniotic fluid
- Cleansing the perineum
- Assessing the perineum

REMEMBER to wash your hands prior to putting the disposable gloves on and AGAIN immediately after you remove the gloves. For further information consult OSHA and CDC guidelines.

contraction is gone), consider the possibility of occiput posterior position (Lipshitz 1990).

4. Assess cervical dilatation and effacement. Cervical dilatation usually progresses at 1.5 cm/hr for multiparas and 1.2 cm/hr for primigravidas. Effacement changes from 0% to 100% during the labor progress. If the cervix becomes edematous and thicker during labor, CPD may be present.

5. Assess fetal position, presentation, and descent. A vaginal examination may identify problems such as breech, transverse brow or face presentation, or occiput posterior.

6. Assess for presence of caput (edema of subcutaneous tissues in the top of the fetal head). An enlarging caput may confuse the examiner because it feels like further descent of the fetal head.

7. Assess descent of the fetal head by determining station.
   Be alert for: the presence of a caput because as the caput enlarges and extends down into the birth canal, it may be mistaken for fetal descent.

8. Assess laboring woman for hydration status, comfort/coping level.

Nursing Diagnoses

- Pain related to inability to relax secondary to labor pattern.
- Risk for ineffective individual coping related to ineffectiveness of breathing techniques to relieve discomfort.

Critical Nursing Interventions

1. Assess labor status by continuous electronic monitoring and monitor labor progress, maternal and fetal status. Compare assessment findings to expected norms.

2. Provide support and comfort measures (see Chapter 3).

3. Monitor oxytocin infusion if ordered by physician (see discussion later in this chapter).

4. Maintain comprehensive charting on maternal-fetal status. Document maternal contraction status (frequency, duration, and intensity of contractions), fetal status (fetal heart rate [FHR] baseline, variability, periodic changes such as accelerations or decelerations), maternal coping and comfort measures used, hydration status, and voiding patterns.

5. Prepare for cesarean birth if indicated.

6. Keep the woman and her partner informed of assessment findings and progress.

7. Review the following critical aspects of the care you have provided.
   - What position does the woman tend to seek? Would any of the following positions work: standing beside the bed and resting on the headrest? sitting on the toilet? using a kneeling or birthing bar? squatting with someone to support her? supported knee to chest? Would ambulation, a shower, or a warm bath help?
   - Have I given support to relaxation and breathing efforts?
   - Are there any other comfort measures available?

Sample Nurse's Charting

Contraction every 2-1/2 minutes, 60 sec duration and of strong intensity. FHR BL 140–148 with two accelerations of 15 bpm with fetal movement in the last 20 minutes. STV present, LTV average. No decelerations present. Voided 200 mL clear amber urine without difficulty. Taking ice chips at will. Skin turgor and mucous membranes indicate adequate hydration. Breathing with contractions but beginning to cry out at the acme. Dozes between contractions but quickly rouses. Asking "Why is it taking so long? Why am I not making progress?" Partner and family asking to speak with physician regarding treatment plan. Call placed to physician and physician to be here in 5 minutes to see patient. P. Gomez, RNC

Evaluation

- The woman will experience a more effective labor pattern.

- The woman has increased comfort and decreased anxiety.

PRECIPITOUS BIRTH

Overview

Precipitous birth is an extremely rapid labor that lasts less than three hours from start to finish. Risks for the mother include lacerations of the cervix, vagina, and/or perineum and postpartal hemorrhage. Fetal/neonatal risks include increased pressure on and in the fetal head and possible cerebral trauma.

Medical Therapy

Close medical monitoring. Obtain previous obstetrical history to identify rapid labor.

Critical Nursing Assessments

1. Assess previous labor history if the woman is a multipara.
2. Assess contraction status. **Be alert for:** contractions that are more frequent than every two minutes and dilatation that progresses faster than normal (more than 1.5 cm per hour).
3. Assess fetal status.

Nursing Diagnoses

- Pain related to accelerated labor pattern.
- Risk for ineffective individual coping related to ineffectiveness of breathing techniques to relieve discomfort.

Critical Nursing Interventions

1. Monitor labor pattern carefully if oxytocin infusion is being used (induction or augmentation).
2. Evaluate fetal response to labor pattern.
3. Provide support and comfort measures for the woman.

4. Assist with the birth of the baby if the physician/certified nurse-midwife is not present.
   - Instruct woman to pant with contractions if fetal head is crowning.
   - Apply gentle pressure against the fetal head to maintain flexion and prevent it from popping out quickly. Support the perineum with the other hand and support the descending head between contractions.
   - Insert two fingers along the back of the fetal neck to check for a nuchal cord. If present, bend the fingers like a fish hook, grasp the cord, and pull it over the baby's head. If the cord cannot be slipped over the head, place two clamps on it and cut between the clamps. Unwind the cord from around the neck.
   - Suction the fetal nares and mouth with a bulb syringe.
   - While requesting the woman to push gently, exert gentle downward pressure on the head and neck to assist in the birth of the anterior shoulder. Then exert gentle upward pressure to assist with the posterior shoulder. Support the rest of the baby's body as it is born.
   - Place newborn on maternal abdomen and dry the baby with soft warm blankets.
   - Check firmness of the uterus. Observe for excessive maternal bleeding.
   - Complete patient records. (For detailed description of assisting at birth see Olds SB, London ML, Ladewig PW: *Maternal-Newborn Nursing: A Family Centered Approach*, 5th ed. Addison-Wesley Nursing, 1996.)

Evaluation

- The woman and her baby are closely monitored during labor and a safe birth occurs.
- The woman feels support and enhanced comfort during labor and birth.

GESTATIONAL AGE-RELATED PROBLEMS

See Table 4–1: Babies with Special Needs in Labor and Birth.

Table 4–1	Babies with Special Needs in Labor and Birth		
Type	Implication for Labor	Treatment	Immediate Nursing Support
Postterm	More likely to have decreased amount of amniotic fluid, so variable decelerations are more likely. Meconium may be present in amniotic fluid.	Biophysical profile (BPP) to assess fetal status. Induction if BPP score decreases, if amniotic fluid volume decreases, or pregnancy reaches 43 wks.	Continuous EFM during labor. At birth, assist physician/CNM with visualization of cord and naso-pharyngeal suctioning if fluid is meconium stained.
Preterm	Stress of labor is difficult for baby. Parents are very concerned about baby. Analgesia may be withheld to avoid depressing the fetus/newborn.	Tocolytic therapy to suppress labor. If not successful, forceps may be used to protect fetal head during vaginal birth, or cesarean birth is performed.	Have pediatrician and nursing support available. Provide respiratory support, temperature stabilization, and rapid assessment of newborn.
Multiple gestation	Vertex-vertex presentation is most common, followed by vertex-breech. Increased risk of prolapsed cord and cord entanglement.	Vaginal birth of vertex-vertex presentation may be possible. Other presentations may be possible with guided ultrasound. Continuous EFM of both babies during labor.	For vaginal birth or cesarean birth, double numbers of personnel are required. Provide respiratory support, temperature stabilization.
Macrosomia (Weight > 4000 grams)	CPD is more likely. Dysfunctional labor due to overstretching of uterine muscle fibers.	If CPD present, then cesarean birth performed.	Baby is more likely to develop hypoglycemia. If shoulder dystocia, assess for shoulder movement, and crepitus over clavicle.

LABOR COMPLICATED BY MALPRESENTATION OR MALPOSITION

See Table 4–2: Impact of Fetal Malpresentation/Position on Birth. (See Figure 4–1 for selected types of fetal malpresentations.)

PROLAPSED UMBILICAL CORD

Overview

Prolapsed cord occurs when the umbilical cord precedes the fetus down the birth canal. Conditions associated with prolapsed cord include breech presentation, transverse lie, contracted pelvic inlet, small fetus, extra long cord, low-lying placenta, hydramnios, and twin gestations. Fetal/neonatal risks include decreased oxygenation and circulation from the compressed umbilical cord and possible fetal distress.

Medical Therapy

Early recognition. Once prolapsed cord is identified, an emergency cesarean birth is usually indicated.

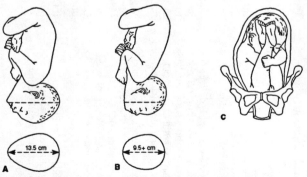

Figure 4–1   Types of malpresentation. A, Brow presentation: The largest anterior-posterior diameter presents to the maternal pelvis. B, Face presentation: Vaginal birth may be possible if the fetal chin is toward the maternal symphysis pubis. C, Breech presentation.

Critical Nursing Assessments

1. Assess woman's present pregnancy for conditions associated with prolapsed cord.

2. Assess FHR. Since cord compression is associated with variable decelerations (decelerations that vary in timing with the contractions), the best method of assessing is by electronic fetal monitoring (EFM). Periodic auscultation may or may not identify a variable deceleration.

3. Assess for presence of cord prolapse.
   Be alert for: the presence of a pulsating, slick cord. (See Figure 4–2.)

Nursing Diagnoses

- Risk for impaired gas exchange in the fetus related to decreased blood flow secondary to compression of the umbilical cord.
- Fear related to unknown outcome.

Critical Nursing Interventions

1. Complete a vaginal examination to check for prolapse of the cord when variable decelerations are noted on EFM tracing.

2. Relieve pressure of the fetal presenting part by leaving the gloved fingers in the vagina and lifting the

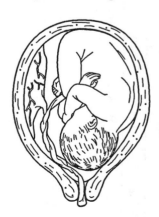

Figure 4–2   Prolapse of the umbilical cord.

Table 4-2	Impact of Fetal Malpresentation/Position on Birth			
Fetal Position	Implication for Labor	Treatment Needed or Anticipated	Nursing Interventions	Impact on Newborn
Occiput posterior	Labor may be longer. Severe back pain may be present.	Forceps or manual rotation at birth may be needed.	Apply sacral pressure. Monitor labor, maternal-fetal status. Assist mother into hands and knees position and instruct her to do pelvic rock. Alternative position would be to put weight on knees and lean over raised head of bed, change position from side to side, squat, and/or sit on a toilet.	If labor is longer, fetus more likely to experience stress. Head is molded.
Brow presentation (See Figure 4-1.)	Labor may be longer.	If CPD is suspected or present, and labor is arrested, then cesarean birth is appropriate.	Monitor labor, maternal-fetal status. Provide support measures. Assist with cesarean birth if indicated.	

Face presentation (See Figure 4-1.)	Risks of CPD and prolonged labor are increased.	If no CPD present and chin (mentum) is anterior, vaginal birth may be possible. If chin is posterior a cesarean birth is necessary.	Monitor labor, maternal-fetal status. Provide support measures. Assist with cesarean birth if indicated.	May develop facial edema during labor. May have edema of throat that compromises breathing.
Breech (See Figure 4-1.)	Labor may be prolonged. Meconium may be expelled in amniotic fluid.	External version may be done at 37–38 weeks and then vaginal birth. If version unsuccessful, cesarean birth is scheduled. Some obstetricians may consider vaginal birth for frank breech.	Monitor labor, maternal-fetal status. Monitor for prolapsed cord.	Newborn has increased risk of mortality, intracranial hemorrhage from traumatic birth of head during vaginal birth. Brachial plexus palsy may occur with vaginal birth.

fetal head off the cord (push fetus up toward the body of the uterus). If possible, place woman in knee-chest or Trendelenburg's position. Maintain the maternal position and pressure on the fetal presenting part until the physician arrives and/or a cesarean birth is accomplished. In some instances, an indwelling bladder catheter may be inserted to fill the bladder with warmed normal saline. The filled bladder places upward pressure on the fetal presenting part and relieves pressure on the cord.

3. Administer oxygen to the mother by face mask at 7–10 L/min.

4. Call for assistance. Other nurses can assist in the preparation of the woman for emergency cesarean birth.

5. Provide information and support to the laboring couple.

6. Review the following critical aspects of the care you have provided.

   • What is the response of the fetal heart rate to the intervention? Has the rate returned to 120–160 range? Is there evidence of variable decelerations on the EFM tracing?

   • Are the variable decelerations lessening in depth? in number?

   • Is the position that I have asked the woman to assume working? Is FHR improving? (See the preceding questions.) Can this position be maintained until a cesarean birth can be accomplished?

   • Is the baby moving much? Are accelerations present?

   • What do I need to protect myself from the woman's bodily fluids? Could a colleague tie a plastic apron around me?

Sample Nurse's Charting

Sterile vaginal exam done to assess dilatation status. Prolapse of the umbilical cord through the cervix and into the vagina. Immediate pressure placed on the fetal vertex. EFM monitor indicates FHR maintained BL of 144–150 from beginning of exam throughout intervention. STV present, LTV average, accelerations of 20 bpm with fetal movement and palpation of fetus. Immediate call placed to Dr. _____ to advise of status. IV of 1000 mL lactated Ringer's started in R wrist after one attempt with 18 gm quikcath. Running at 125 mL/hr. 16Fr indwelling Foley catheter inserted. Abdominal-perineal prep done. To surgery for emergency cesarean section. Continuous pressure placed on fetal vertex through the vagina until birth. Permit signed by husband. P. Gomez, RNC

AMNIOTIC FLUID-RELATED COMPLICATION: HYDRAMNIOS

Overview

Hydramnios occurs when there is over 2000 mL of amniotic fluid in the amniotic sac. The exact cause of hydramnios is unknown; however, it often occurs in cases of major congenital anomalies. Maternal risks include shortness of breath and edema in the lower extremities from compression of the vena cava. The fetus/neonate has an increased risk of mortality because of associated fetal malformations (more prevalent with hydramnios) and increased incidence of preterm birth. Malpresentation is more likely, as is prolapse of the cord.

Medical Therapy

1. **Provide supportive therapy.** Assess fundal size and monitor growth throughout pregnancy. Complete ultrasound examinations to determine presence of anomalies.

2. **Decrease amount of amniotic fluid.** In some instances, an amniocentesis may be done to remove fluid in order to reduce the risk of preterm labor.

Critical Nursing Assessments

1. Assess woman's history for other associated problems such as diabetes, Rh sensitization, fetal malformations, or multiple gestation.

2. Assess FHR. It may be more difficult to auscultate the FHR because of the increased amount of fluid. Placement of the EFM may also be more difficult because of the size of the maternal abdomen. **Be alert for:** the presence of variable decelerations that may indicate prolapse of the cord.

3. Assess maternal blood pressure (BP) and respiratory rate (weight of the uterus can compromise maternal circulation). If compression of the vena cava occurs, hypotension, rapid pulse, pallor, and dyspnea may be noted. Vena caval compression is more likely when the pregnant woman is lying on her back.

4. Assess for fetal malpresentation-malposition by sterile vaginal examination to determine fetal presenting part.

Nursing Diagnoses

- Risk for alteration in gas exchange related to pressure on the diaphragm secondary to hydramnios.
- Fear related to unknown outcome of the pregnancy.

Critical Nursing Interventions

1. Position woman on left or right side.

2. Monitor maternal and fetal status frequently. Follow NAACOG recommended guidelines for labor (see Table 3–5 on page 81). Because of increased incidence of fetal problems, continuous EFM may be warranted.

3. Monitor amount of amniotic fluid lost, and characteristics of fluid. **Be alert for:** presence of meconium in the fluid (may be associated with fetal stress/distress).

Evaluation

- Maternal and fetal status remains stable with BP, pulse, respirations, and FHR in normal range.
- Woman's questions and fears are addressed.

AMNIOTIC FLUID-RELATED COMPLICATION: OLIGOHYDRAMNIOS

Overview

In oligohydramnios, the amount of amniotic fluid is severely reduced and concentrated. The exact cause is unknown; however, it is found in cases of postmaturity, with intrauterine growth retardation (IUGR) secondary to placental insufficiency, and in fetal conditions associated with renal and urinary malfunction.

Because the amount of amniotic fluid is reduced, the umbilical cord has less fluid to float in. The umbilical cord is more likely to be compressed (indicated by variable decelerations), and the blood flow to the fetus is reduced. Maternal risks include dysfunctional labor. Fetal risks include fetal hypoxia associated with umbilical cord compression. If oligohydramnios has been present throughout the gestation, the fetus may have pulmonary hypoplasia.

Medical Therapy

1. **Identify presence of oligohydramnios.** Oligohydramnios is usually identified by serial ultrasound examinations during pregnancy. During labor, an amnioinfusion (infusion of warmed saline solution) may be done to decrease the risk of cord compression.

2. **Monitor fetal status.** Monitor fetus with biophysical profiles.

Critical Nursing Assessments

1. Assess results of any prenatal testing that indicate decreased amniotic fluid volume (ultrasound exam with notations of decreased volume, or biophysical profile (BPP) score that is decreased because of diminished amniotic fluid volume.

2. Assess FHR. **Be alert for:** variable decelerations.

3. If membranes rupture, note color and amount of fluid (will be assessed as scant, small, moderate, or large amount), and assess for the presence of meconium.

Nursing Diagnoses

- Risk for impaired gas exchange related to pressure on the umbilical cord secondary to decreased amniotic fluid.
- Fear related to unknown outcome of pregnancy.

Critical Nursing Interventions

1. Monitor maternal and fetal status on a frequent basis. Watch for maternal hypotension, anxiety, or tension (may be associated with decreased placental-fetal perfusion).

2. Be alert for presence of variable decelerations and decreased variability.

3. Encourage woman to maintain side-lying position while in bed.

4. Assist with amnioinfusion if done.

Evaluation

- The woman and her partner understand the condition, need for monitoring, and possible associated problems.
- The woman and her baby are monitored closely throughout the labor and birth.

AMNIOTIC FLUID EMBOLISM

Overview

An amniotic fluid embolism is a catastrophic event that occurs when a small amount of amniotic fluid enters the maternal blood stream. The bolus of amniotic fluid moves through the maternal circulation, through the right atrium and ventricle, and then into the pulmonary circulation. The sequence of events is thought to include transient pulmonary arterial spasm producing hypoxia with left ventricular and pulmonary capillary injury. This is followed by left ventricular failure and the acute development of adult respiratory distress syndrome (ARDS). The etiology of the coagulopathy that also occurs is unknown (Niswander & Evans 1991).

Maternal mortality rate is 80% (Niswander & Evans 1991). Fetal hypoxia/anoxia occurs as the mother experiences respiratory difficulty or respiratory arrest.

Medical Therapy

Emergency support measures. Immediate, intensive care to support circulatory and respiratory systems is required. Oxygen is administered by mask or positive pressure. The mother may need to be intubated, and numerous IV lines are placed. Central hemodynamic monitoring lines are necessary to monitor pressures and make treatment decisions. IV fluids are given for hypotension, and dopamine may be required to maintain maternal blood pressure. Coagulation studies are completed to monitor the development of consumption coagulopathy (DIC) and to monitor treatment. Continuous EFM is necessary to monitor fetal status (Niswander & Evans 1991).

Critical Nursing Assessments

1. Assess for associated factors such as multiparity, hydramnios, tumultuous labor (contractions with frequency of less than two minutes and strong intensity. This type of labor may occur naturally or be associated with intravenous oxytocin administration).

2. Assess maternal vital signs. **Be alert for:** signs of respiratory distress or any statement from the mother that she is experiencing difficulty breathing. The amount of difficulty seems to vary according to the amount of amniotic fluid in the bolus. A large bolus will cause immediate, overwhelming respiratory problems.

3. Assess FHR. Evaluate FHR rate, variability, and presence of decelerations.

4. Assess labor progress and identify hypertonic labor patterns (contractions more frequent than every two minutes and/or duration greater than 90 seconds with strong intensity).

Nursing Diagnoses

- Risk for impaired gas exchange related to cardio-pulmonary collapse.
- Fear related to unknown outcome of the complication.

Critical Nursing Interventions

1. Continue to monitor and evaluate maternal-fetal status.

2. If respiratory difficulties occur, quickly assess, provide oxygen, call for emergency assistance, and provide respiratory and cardiac support until assistance arrives. Start one or two peripheral IV lines and assist with emergency measures. Have one nurse note the type and administration time of all medications. Monitor fetal status at all times.

3. Complete client records. Nurses' notes need to reflect the time symptoms began and what the signs and symptoms were, the actions taken and response of the client. Continuing assessments are also documented.

4. Prepare for emergency cesarean birth.

Evaluation

- The mother and baby are monitored carefully.
- Emergency measures are instituted immediately.

ABRUPTIO PLACENTA IN THE INTRAPARTAL AREA

Overview

When a woman is admitted to the intrapartal area and she is bleeding, it is important to complete assessments quickly and to differentiate between many possible causes of the bleeding. Knowledge of the type of bleeding and the presence or absence of pain may assist in this differentiation (see Table 4–3). The maternal mortality

Table 4–3	Characteristics of Placenta Previa and Abruptio Placenta	
Placenta Previa	**Abruptio Placenta**
Bright red bleeding	May be bright red or dark red in color or no bleeding may be apparent if abruption is concealed
No pain	May have no pain if abruption was on margin of placenta and has now resolved
May have history of painless, bright red bleeding	May have pain if abruption is central (behind placenta). If contractions are present, may have increased tonus of uterus and poor uterine relaxation between contractions. Uterus may be "boardlike"

rate is approximately 6%. Other complications include hemorrhage and development of DIC. Fetal/neonatal risks include anemia and hypoxia.

Medical Therapy

1. **Mild abruption** (vaginal bleeding absent or external bleeding of less than 100 mL). The labor can continue and vaginal birth is anticipated.

2. **Moderate abruption** (vaginal bleeding absent or from 100–500 mL) and **severe abruption** (vaginal bleeding absent or greater than 500 mL) require continuous monitoring of the mother and fetus, monitoring and treatment of shock, possibly an amniotomy and oxytocin infusion to augment labor or begin labor, evaluation of coagulation, blood replacement, and possible cesarean section.

3. **Method of birth.** Cesarean birth is indicated when: (1) fetal distress develops and a vaginal birth is not imminent, (2) the fetus is alive and a severe abruption occurs, (3) hemorrhage becomes severe and threatens the life of the mother, and (4) labor is not progressing.

Critical Nursing Assessments

1. Assess maternal history for associated factors (pregnancy-induced hypertension [PIH], high multiparity, trauma, use of illicit drugs such as cocaine or crack).

2. Assess type and amount of bleeding. Pads may be weighed to assess blood loss more accurately (1 gram equals 1 mL). Hemorrhage of 500 mL or more increases chance of fetal death. Vaginal bleeding is present in 80% of abruptions and is absent (concealed) in other 20% (Niswander & Evans 1991).

3. Assess whether pain is present. Is pain associated with uterine contractions? Is there pain between contractions (feels as if the uterus stays tight and does not relax). Are there tender areas over the uterus? Pain is present in most women with abruptio placenta. The pain is usually of sudden onset, is constant, and is localized to the uterus or the lower back (Niswander & Evans 1991).

4. Assess uterine contractions. What is frequency, duration, intensity, and what is resting tone between contractions? (Abruptio is associated with a rising uterine tone baseline.)

5. Assess size of uterus. If bleeding is concealed, the uterus may be filling with blood and the fundus will rise.

6. Assess labor progress (vaginal examination for cervical dilatation, effacement, and fetal station). Abruption may be associated with precipitous birth.

7. Assess maternal vital signs (BP, pulse, respirations) and fetal status (by EFM).

8. Assess laboratory studies (hemoglobin, hematocrit, DIC screen).

Nursing Diagnoses

- Fluid volume deficit related to hypovolemia secondary to excessive blood loss.
- Anxiety related to concern for own personal status and the baby's safety.

Critical Nursing Interventions

1. Monitor maternal status. Be alert for beginning signs of shock (decreased BP, increased pulse, increased respirations).

2. Monitor fetal status. Be alert for FHR baseline changes and late decelerations with decreased variability.

3. Monitor amount of blood loss. Measure blood loss. Wear disposable gloves when handling blood-soaked items or while cleansing blood from woman.

4. Carefully monitor labor status. Be alert for increased uterine tonus, which may be exhibited by increased frequency of contractions (< two minutes), increased intensity, incomplete uterine relaxation between contractions, tenderness of the uterine fundus, and a rising baseline of EFM monitor strip.

5. Monitor urine output. Urine output is reflective of circulatory status. Urine output needs to be at least 30 mL/hr. An indwelling bladder catheter will assist in monitoring urine output accurately. Amount of output is measured every one to four hours, depending on severity of bleeding.

6. Monitor size of abdomen. Measurement of abdominal girth may be ordered. If it is, place measuring tape under woman, bring around to the front and over the umbilicus. Use either the upper or lower edge of the umbilicus and, for consistency, consider making marks on the maternal abdomen with felt-tip pen to ensure consistent placement of the tape in each measurement.

7. Monitor oxytocin if it is being administered. See discussion of induction of labor later in this chapter.

8. Monitor laboratory studies. Be alert for development of consumption coagulopathy (DIC) as evidenced by decreasing platelets and fibrinogen and increased fibrin split products. (See Table 4–4.)

9. Monitor oxygen status by pulse oximetry (pulse oximetry needs to be 90 or above). If reading is below 90, administer oxygen by face mask at 7–10 L/min.

10. Monitor fluid and blood replacement.

**Table 4–4   Laboratory Findings Associated
with DIC**

Lab Test	Normal Value	Value in DIC
Partial thromboplastin	60–70 sec	Prolonged
Platelets	150,000–400,000 μL	Decreased
Fibrinogen	200–400 mg/dL	Decreased
Fibrin degradation products (also called fibrin split products or fibrin)	2–10 μg/mL	Increased

11. Monitor for signs of decreased platelet count such as purpura, petechiae, bruising, hematemesis, rectal bleeding.

12. Prepare for cesarean if birth not imminent.

13. Follow body substance isolation and CDC precautions at all times of exposure to bodily fluids.

14. Review the following critical aspects of the care you have provided.

   - Are the woman's vital signs stable? Are they responding in an anticipated way to the medical therapy? What does the woman say about her condition? Is she anxious?
   - Is the amount of bleeding increasing? What are the measured amounts of blood loss? Is there bleeding from any other site?
   - Is the uterus becoming more tender, more sensitive?
   - Is there a rising uterine resting tone?
   - Is there a better position to place the woman in to maximize circulation and comfort?
   - What other information can I provide?
   - Has there been a change in her consciousness level?

Sample Nurse's Charting

Uterine contractions every 3 min, 60 sec duration and strong intensity. Uterus relaxes between contractions. Patient reports slight tenderness in the upper uterine fundus on the right when palpated. FHR 140–146, STV diminished, LTV decreased, no accelerations with fetal movement. Deceleration of 15 bpm lasting 15 sec begins just after acme of each contraction. O_2 per face mask at 8 L/min. Patient lying on left side. BP stable at 112/70. Admitting BP 114/72. Pulse 80 and regular. 100 cc dark red vaginal bleeding present on Chux in last hour. Patient breathing with contractions and relaxing well with encouragement. Partner provides continuous, ongoing support. P. Gomez, RNC

Evaluation

- The woman and her baby have a safe labor and birth without further complications.
- The woman and family verbalize understanding of reasons for medical therapy and risks.

PLACENTA PREVIA IN THE INTRAPARTAL PERIOD

Overview

Placenta previa may occur as a low placental implantation, a partial or marginal previa, or a complete previa. Maternal risks include hemorrhage and possible complications of emergency cesarean birth. Fetal/neonatal risks include anemia and, if bleeding occurs, hypoxia.

Medical Therapy

Management. Obtain diagnosis from ultrasound examination. If complete previa, gestation > 37 weeks, and documented fetal maturity, schedule cesarean birth. If marginal placenta previa, labor and vaginal birth may be possible.

Critical Nursing Assessments

1. Assess type and amount of bleeding (as in previous section on abruption).
2. Assess maternal vital signs and fetal status.

3. Assess labor progress (uterine contraction frequency, duration, and intensity; fetal descent).

4. Assess laboratory findings.

Nursing Diagnoses

- Risk for altered tissue perfusion related to blood loss.
- Risk for impaired fetal gas exchange related to decreased blood volume and hypotension.

Critical Nursing Interventions

1. Monitor bleeding. Weigh all absorbent pads to determine amount of blood loss.

2. Monitor maternal vital signs for signs of shock.

3. Monitor FHR for evidence of normality (baseline stable, short-term variability (STV) present and average long-term variability (LTV), no periodic decelerations or early decelerations). Note signs of possible fetal problems such as rising or falling baseline, decreased variability, late and/or variable decelerations.

4. Monitor laboratory studies. **Be alert for:** evidence of decreasing hemoglobin and hematocrit. **Note:** Coagulation problems are not as common with placenta previa as with abruptio placenta?

5. Administer and monitor IV fluids and blood replacement.

6. Monitor oxygen status. If vital signs unstable or questionable, monitor pulse oximetry. If pulse oximetry is below 90, administer oxygen by face mask at 7–10 L/min. Continue to monitor pulse oximetry.

Evaluation

- The hemorrhage ceases and any hypovolemia is corrected as indicated by normal blood studies and normal maternal vital signs.
- . Any signs of fetal distress are recognized promptly, and corrective measures are begun.

- The woman and her baby have a safe labor and birth without further complications for the mother or child.
- The woman and family verbalize understanding of risks and reasons for medical therapy.

DIABETES MELLITUS IN THE INTRAPARTAL PERIOD

Overview

Diabetes affects the labor process in a variety of ways. Insulin/glucose balance is affected by the expenditure of energy during labor. The method of birth will be influenced by assessment of the fetal size. A large fetus (> 4500 gr or a fetus larger than the maternal pelvis) will be born by cesarean.

Effect of Diabetes	Medical Therapy	Nursing Interventions
Alteration of insulin/glucose balance	Schedule cesarean in early AM. Advise client to have her usual evening insulin dose, evening meal, and snack.	Monitor blood glucose by finger-stick at evening meal and at bedtime.
		Be watchful for signs and symptoms of hypo- or hyperglycemia.
		Expect precipitous drop in insulin requirements after birth.
	If client is laboring, monitor blood glucose by hourly fingersticks and administration of insulin and IV fluids. Maintain glucose control at < 100 mg/dL.	Assist with finger-sticks. Adjust IV fluids per physician order. Administer insulin per physician order.

Effect of Diabetes	Medical Therapy	Nursing Interventions
Increased incidence of large fetus	Estimate fetal size.	Maintain mother in side-lying position.
		Monitor FHR by EFM.
		Evaluate labor progress carefully to watch for failure to progress or evidence of CPD.
		Evaluate EFM tracing for late deceleration and/or decreased variability.
Increased incidence of congenital anomalies		Assess newborn for signs of congenital problems.
Acceleration of fetal lung maturity	Determine fetal lung maturity prior to labor.	Have resuscitation equipment and personnel available at birth.

PREGNANCY-INDUCED HYPERTENSION IN THE INTRAPARTAL PERIOD

Overview

The woman with pregnancy-induced hypertension needs to be watched closely in the intrapartal area. Her blood pressure may increase with the stress of labor. Hyper-irritability of the central nervous system (CNS) may affect the woman's ability to cope with the labor process.

Effect of labor	Medical Therapy	Nursing Interventions
Possible increase of blood pressure	IV magnesium sulfate therapy	Start and monitor IV magnesium sulfate therapy by infusion pump.

Effect of Labor	Medical Therapy	Nursing Interventions
Possible increase of blood pressure *(continued)*		Check BP, pulse, respirations, patellar and brachial reflexes, and urine output at least hourly (more often if maternal condition requires).
		Remember therapeutic magnesium sulfate level is from 4–8 mg/dL.
		Loss of patellar reflex is the earliest sign of magnesium toxicity; this occurs at about 8–10 mg/dL.
		Respiratory and cardiac arrest may occur if magnesium levels rise further. See Drug Guide: Magnesium Sulfate ($MgSO_4$).
Stress of labor on fetus	Evaluate fetal status.	Maintain continuous EFM. Assess tracing frequently for late decelerations or decreased variability.

INDUCTION OF LABOR

Overview

Labor may be induced when diabetes, PIH, premature rupture of membranes (PROM), postterm pregnancy, intrauterine growth retardation (IUGR), and intrauterine fetal death (IUFD) are present. The most frequent methods of induction are amniotomy, intravenous administration of oxytocin, or both. Prostaglandin E_2 is currently being used for labor priming (softening of the cervix) at term but is not used to induce labor at that time.

Cervical readiness for induction can be assessed by determining a Bishop's score. A score of at least 9 is usually associated with a successful induction (see Table 4–5).

For oxytocin induction 1000 mL of solution (such as lactated Ringer's) is started IV by a large-bore plastic IV catheter (18 or 20 gauge). Ten units of pitocin are added to a second 1000-mL bottle of IV fluid (second bottle needs to match the other primary IV). The IV containing the pitocin is the secondary bottle and this bottle is administered via an infusion pump. (See Drug Guide: Oxytocin [Pitocin] for further information.)

Maternal risks include water intoxication; rapid labor and birth; cervical, vaginal, and/or perineal lacerations. Fetal/neonatal risks include rapid intracranial pressure changes if rapid labor and birth occur, possible decreased placental-fetal circulation if labor pattern is overstimulated.

Critical Nursing Assessments

1. Assess woman's knowledge and understanding regarding the induction procedure, associated nursing care, risks and benefits.

2. Assess for any contraindications to the induction procedure (client refusal, presence of placenta previa, abnormal fetal presentation, prolapsed cord, presenting part above the inlet, active genital herpes infection, CPD, severe fetal stress or distress, presence of FHR late decelerations).

3. Assess maternal vital signs to provide a baseline for further assessments.

4. Assess fetal heart rate characteristics after obtaining a 20-minute EFM strip. Assess FHR for reassuring characteristics (baseline between 120 and 160, STV present, LTV average, accelerations with fetal movement, no late or variable decelerations present).

5. Assess maternal vital signs, contraction pattern and characteristics, and cervical dilatation and fetal response to IV oxytocin once infusion has begun and with each planned increase in the infusion rate.

6. Assess maternal physiologic and psychologic response to uterine contractions.

Nursing Diagnoses

- Knowledge deficit related to information about induction procedure.
- Risk for altered placental tissue perfusion related to potential hypertonic contraction pattern.

Critical Nursing Interventions

1. Provide information to meet knowledge needs of woman and her partner.

2. Administer oxytocin as a secondary infusion and increase infusion pump rate according to agency protocol.

3. Monitor contraction and cervical dilatation pattern and EFM tracing. If contractions occur more frequently than every two minutes, decrease the infusion rate. If fetal stress occurs (decreasing variability, decreasing baseline or presence of late decelerations), discontinue oxytocin infusion and infuse primary IV solution, institute supportive nursing care (assist to side-lying position, monitor for hypotension, and initiate oxygen) and notify physician/CNM.

4. Monitor maternal vital signs, contraction pattern, cervical dilatation status, and EFM tracing on a periodic basis and prior to any increase of oxytocin. (See Drug Guide 7: Oxytocin [Pitocin] for additional information.)

5. Provide supportive nursing measures to increase maternal comfort.

6. Advocate for the laboring woman when she requests analgesia or anesthesia block.

7. Advise CNM/physician of maternal/fetal condition on a frequent basis.

8. Carefully evaluate need for changes in the infusion rate of oxytocin (increase, decrease, or maintain rate) once active labor pattern.

Evaluation

- Woman verbalizes understanding of the medication utilized, the need to take vital signs frequently, and the need for continuing fetal monitoring to evaluate contractions and fetal response.

- Woman experiences contraction pattern that remains within normal limits.

Table 4-5 Prelabor Status Evaluation Scoring System*

	Assigned Value			
Factor	**0**	**1**	**2**	**3**
Cervical dilatation	Closed	1–2 cm	3–4 cm	5 cm or more
Cervical effacement	0%–30%	40%–50%	60%–70%	80% or more
Fetal station	–3	–2	–1, 0	+1, or lower
Cervical consistency	Firm	Moderate	Soft	
Cervical position	Posterior	Midposition	Anterior	

*Modified from Bishop EH; Pelvic scoring for elective induction. *Obstet Gynecol* 1964; 24:266.

OBSTETRIC PROCEDURE: EXTERNAL VERSION

Procedure Overview

Version is done to change the fetal presentation from breech to cephalic. It is usually scheduled in the 38th week of pregnancy but may be done in the 39th or 40th.

Critical Nursing Assessments

1. Assess the mother for presence of contraindications (nonreactive nonstress test [NST], evidence of CPD, multiple gestation, oligohydramnios, ruptured amniotic membranes, and placenta previa).

2. Assess maternal BP, pulse and respirations, and fetal heart rate (establish presence of reassuring characteristics: FHR baseline between 120–160, presence of short-term variability and average long-term variability, absence of late or variable decelerations).

Nursing Diagnoses

- Knowledge deficit related to procedure and possible complications

Critical Nursing Interventions

1. Monitor maternal BP and pulse prior to the version and every five minutes during the procedure.

2. Administer tocolytic per physician order.

3. Monitor fetal heart rate continuously during the version.

4. Provide support to the woman and her partner.

5. Provide information regarding the version.

6. Determine woman's Rh status. If she is Rh negative, obstetrician will probably order mini-dose of RhoGam.

7. Provide teaching regarding signs and symptoms to watch for.

Evaluation

- The version is accomplished successfully and no complications have occurred.
- The woman is knowledgeable regarding possible complications.

OBSTETRIC PROCEDURE: FORCEPS-ASSISTED BIRTH

Procedure Overview

Forceps may be used for rotation of the fetus when there is a persistent posterior position or transverse arrest (anterior-posterior diameters of the fetal head remain transverse in the maternal pelvis), and for traction to assist birth. Maternal risks include laceration of the cervix, vagina, or perineum; or hematoma. Fetal/neonatal risks include possible stress, facial edema, and/or bruising.

Critical Nursing Assessments

1. Assess maternal ability to relax perineal muscles during forceps application and use.
2. Assess maternal and fetal status (vital signs) and contraction pattern.

Nursing Diagnoses

- Knowledge deficit related to procedure and possible complications
- Ineffective individual coping related to unexpected labor progress and use of procedure

Critical Nursing Interventions

1. Monitor woman's comfort/coping level.
2. Monitor uterine contractions and inform physician of presence of contractions.
3. Monitor FHR after each contraction or continuously by EFM.
4. Provide information and support to the woman.

Evaluation

- Mother and baby have experienced no complications.
- Mother and partner understand procedure and possible complications.

OBSTETRIC PROCEDURE: VACUUM EXTRACTION

Procedure Overview

The vacuum extractor is composed of a suction cup attached to a suction device (bottle). The suction cup is placed against the fetal occiput, and traction can be applied by the obstetrician to assist the birth. The maternal risks are similar to those in the use of forceps. Fetal/neonatal risks are similar except that facial edema or bruising does not occur; instead, a caput (called a chignon) forms under the suction cup.

Nursing assessments, diagnoses, interventions, and evaluation are similar to those in forceps-assisted birth.

REFERENCES

Lipshitz J: Failure to progress in labor. In: Rivlin ME, Morrison JC, Bates GW (editors): *Manual of Clinical Problems in Obstetrics and Gynecology.* Boston: Little, Brown, 1990.

Niswander KR, Evans A: *Manual of Obstetrics.* Boston: Little, Brown, 1991.

CHAPTER 5

The Normal Newborn

At the moment of birth, numerous physiologic adaptations begin to take place in the newborn's body. Because of these dramatic changes, the newborn requires close observation to determine how smoothly she or he is making the transition to extrauterine life. The newborn also requires care that enhances her or his chances of making the transition successfully.

Two broad goals of nursing care during this period are to promote the physical well-being of the newborn and to promote the establishment of a well-functioning family unit. The first goal is met by providing comprehensive care to the newborn while he or she is in the nursery. The second goal is met by teaching parents how to care for their new baby and by supporting their parenting efforts so that they feel confident and competent.

TRANSITIONAL PERIOD

The transitional period involves three periods, called the first period of reactivity, sleep phase, and second period of reactivity. The characteristics of each period demonstrate the newborn's progression to independent functioning.

First Period of Reactivity

This period lasts from birth to 30–60 minutes after birth.

Characteristics

1. The newborn's vital signs are as follows: apical pulse rate between 120–150 bpm (but may be as

high as 180 bpm) and irregular in rhythm. Respiratory rate between 30 and 60 breaths/minute, irregular, and some may be labored, with nasal flaring, expiratory grunting, and retractions.

2. Color fluctuates from pale pink to cyanotic.

3. Bowel sounds are absent and the baby usually does not void or stool during this period.

4. The newborn has minimal amounts of mucus at this time, a rigorous cry, and strong suck reflex. Special tip: During this period of time, the newborn's eyes are open more than they will be again for days. It is an excellent time for the attachment process to begin as the newborn is able to maintain eye contact for long periods of time.

Care needs specific to first period of reactivity

1. Assess and monitor heart rate and respirations q30 min for the first four hours after birth.

2. Keep baby warm (axillary or skin probe temperature between 36.5C to 37C [97.7F–98.6F]) with warmed blankets or overhead warming lights.

3. Couple mother and baby together skin to skin to facilitate attachment.

4. Delay instillation of eye prophylactic for first hour to promote newborn-parent interaction.

Sleep Phase

The sleep phase begins from 30–60 minutes after birth and lasts from four to six hours after birth.

Characteristics

1. As the baby moves into the sleep phase, the heart rate may remain irregular until sleep occurs. While asleep, the respiratory rate increases and the apical pulse rate ranges from 120–140 bpm.

2. Skin color stabilizes, some acrocyanosis may be present.

Care needs specific to sleep phase The baby doesn't respond to external stimuli. Mother and father can still enjoy holding and cuddling their baby.

Second Period of Reactivity

The second period of reactivity lasts from 4–6 hours of age to 8–12 hours of age.

Characteristics

1. Baby has intense sensitivity to internal and environmental stimuli. Apical pulse ranges from 120–160 bpm and can vary from this range from bradycardia (< 120 bpm) to tachycardia (> 160 bpm). Respiratory rate (RR) is 30–60 breaths/minute with periods of more rapid respirations, but they remain unlabored (no nasal flaring or retractions).

2. Skin color fluctuates from pink or ruddy to cyanotic with periods of mottling.

3. Baby often voids and passes meconium during this period.

4. Mucous secretions increases and the baby may gag on secretions. Sucking reflex is again strong, and baby may be very active.

Care needs specific to second period of reactivity

1. Close observation of newborn for possible choking on the excessive mucus normally present. Use bulb syringe to remove mucus and teach parents how to use the bulb syringe.

2. Observe for any episode of apnea and initiate methods of stimulation if needed (stroke baby's back, turn baby to side, etc).

3. Assess baby's interest in and ability to feed (no choking or gagging during feeding, no vomiting of feeding in unchanged form).

Additional Assessments and Interventions in the Transitional Period

In these first few hours of life, the nurse will accomplish the following:

1. Monitor newborn vital signs. See Table 5–1 for summary of normal findings.
2. Weigh the newborn, and measure length, head, and

Table 5–1   Key Signs of Newborn Transition

Pulse: 120–150 beats/min
    During sleep as low as 100 beats/min; if crying, up to 180 beats/min

Respirations: 30–60 respirations/min
    Predominantly diaphragmatic but synchronous with abdominal movements

Temperature: Axillary: 36.5C–37C (97.7F–98.6F)
    Skin: 36C–36.5C (96.8F–97.7F)

Dextrostix: greater than 45 mg %

Hematocrit: less than 65%–70% central venous sample

Blood pressure: 90–60/45–40 mm Hg

Table 5–2   Newborn Weight and Measurements

Weight
Average: 3405 grams (7 lb, 8 oz)
Range: 2500–4000 grams (s lb, 8 oz to 8 lb, 13 oz)
Weight is influenced by racial origin and maternal age and size

Length
Average: 50 cm (20 in)
Range: 45–55 cm (18–22 in)

Head Circumference
Average: 32–37 cm (12 1/2–14 1/2 in)
Approximately 2 cm (about 1 inch) larger than chest circumference

---

chest circumference (see Table 5–2 and Figure 5–1). To determine length, place the newborn flat on her/his back with legs extended as much as possible. Hold the head still at the top of the measuring tape and gently stretch the legs downward toward the bottom of the tape (see Figure 5–2). To measure head circumference place the tape over the most prominent part of the occiput and bring it around above the eyebrows (see Figure 5–3). The circumference of the head is approximately 2 cm greater than the circumference of the chest at birth.

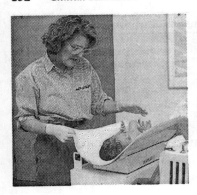

Figure 5–1
Weighing of new-borns. The scale is balanced before each weight, with the protective pad in place. The care giver's hand is poised above the infant as a safety measure.

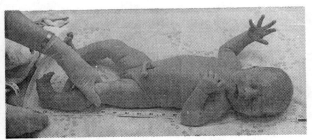

Figure 5–2   Measuring the length of a newborn.

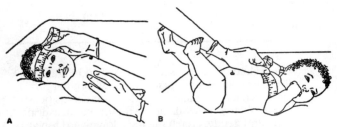

A   **B**

Figure 5–3   Obtaining newborn measurements.
A, Measuring the head circumference of the newborn. The tape is placed on the occiput and then brought around and placed just above the eyebrows. B, Measuring the chest circumference of the newborn. The tape is placed over the lower edge of the scapula and brought around to the front and placed over the nipple line.

To obtain chest circumference, place the tape measure at the lower edge of the scapulas and bring it around anteriorly over the nipple line.

3. Complete gestational age assessment of the newborn. The nurse needs to complete this assessment during the first four hours of life so that age-related problems can be identified. Clinical gestational age assessment tools have two components: external physical characteristics and neuromuscular status.

   Physical characteristics (with the exception of sole creases) can be assessed over the first 24 hours. Neuromuscular development may be influenced by the newborn's unstable nervous system or labor and birth events. It can be assessed in the first 24 hours; however, if the findings drastically differ from the gestational age determined by looking at physical characteristics, the assessment may be repeated after 24 hours (see Table 5–3).

   Method of assessment Use Estimation of Gestational Age by Maturity Rating (Figure 5–4). Assess each of the factors listed and assign a score of 0 to 4 for each one. It is helpful to circle the results for each assessment.

Table 5–3   Characteristics of Gestational Age Assessment

Physical Characteristics	Neuromuscular Characteristics
Characteristics of skin	Posture
Amount of lanugo	Square window (wrist)
Sole creases	Arm recoil
Amount of breast tissue	Popliteal angle
Cartilaginous development of the ear	Scarf sign
Male: testicular descent and rugae on scrotum OR	Heel to ear
Female: labial development	

NEWBORN MATURITY RATING & CLASSIFICATION

ESTIMATION OF GESTATIONAL AGE BY MATURITY RATING
Symbols: X - 1st Exam O - 2nd Exam

NEUROMUSCULAR MATURITY

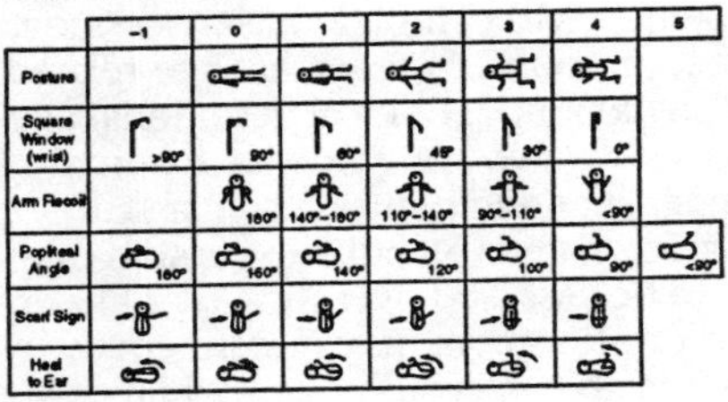

Gestation by Dates ________ wks

Birth Date ________ Hour ________ am pm

APGAR ________ 1 min ________ 5

MATURITY RATING

score	weeks
-10	20
-5	22
0	24
5	26
10	28
15	30
20	32
25	34
30	36
35	38
40	40
45	42
50	44

PHYSICAL MATURITY

Skin	sticky friable transparent	gelatinous red, translucent	smooth pink, visible veins	superficial peeling &/or rash, few veins	cracking pale areas rare veins	parchment deep cracking no vessels	leathery cracked wrinkled
Lanugo	none	sparse	abundent	thinning	bald areas	mostly bald	
Planter Surface	heel-toe 40-50mm:-1 <40mm:-2	>50mm no crease	faint red marks	anterior transverse crease only	creases ant. 2/3	creases over entire sole	
Breast	imperceptible	barely perceptible	flat areola no bud	stippled areola 1–2mm bud	raised areola 3–4mm bud	full areola 5–10mm bud	
Eye/Ear	lids fused loosely:-1 tightly:-2	lids opén pinna flat stays folded	sl. curved pinna; soft; slow recoil	well curved pinna; soft but ready recoil	formed & firm instant recoil	thick cartilage ear stiff	
Genitals male	scrotum flat, smooth	scrotum empty faint rugae	testes in upper canal rare rugae	testes descending few rugae	testes down good rugae	testes pendulous deep rugae	
Genitals female	clitoris prominent labia flat	prominent clitoris small labia minora	prominent clitoris enlarging minora	majora & minora equally prominent	majora large minora small	majora cover clitoris & minora	

SCORING SECTION

	1st Exam = X	2nd Exam = 0
Estimating Gest Age by Maturity Rating	________ Weeks	________ Weeks
Time of Exam	Date ________ Hour ________ am pm	Date ________ Hour ________ am pm
Age at Exam	________ Hours	________ Hours
Signature of Examiner	________ ________ M.D.	________ ________ M.D.

Figure 5–4 Newborn maturity rating and classification. (From Ballard JL, et al: A simplified assessment of gestational age. Classification of the low-birth-weight infant. In: Klaus MH, **Pediatr Res** ***1977; 11:374. Figure adapted from Sweet AY, Fanaroff AA:*** **Care of the High-Risk Infant.** ***Philadelphia: Saunders, 1977, p47.)***

Physical characteristics

a. **Skin** in the preterm neonate appears thin and transparent, with veins prominent over the abdomen early in gestation. As term approaches, the skin appears opaque because of increased subcutaneous tissue. Disappearance of the protective vernix caseosa promotes skin desquamation (peeling).

b. **Lanugo,** a fine hair covering, decreases as gestational age increases. The amount of lanugo is greatest at 28–30 weeks and then disappears, first from the face, then from the trunk and extremities.

c. **Sole (plantar creases)** needs to be assessed within 12 hours of birth because after this the skin of the foot begins drying and superficial creases disappear. Development of sole creases begins at the top of the sole and proceeds downward toward the heel.

d. **Areola** is inspected and the breast bud tissue is gently palpated to determine the size. It is important to place your index and middle finger over this tissue and roll over the breast bud to estimate the size, rather than pinching the tissue. Another method of measuring involves placing a ruler just above the breast bud tissue for more accurate measurement. Most experienced nurses have completed the assessment often enough that they can estimate the size very accurately.

e. **Ear form and cartilage** change throughout gestation. By 36 weeks some cartilage and slight incurving of upper pinna are present, and the pinna springs back slowly when folded.
To assess, observe ear form and then fold pinna of the ear forward against the side of the head, release it, and observe the results.

f. **Genitals** change in appearance during gestation because of the amount of subcutaneous fat present. **Female genitals** at 30–32 weeks have a prominent clitoris, and the labia majora are small and widely separated. At 36–40 weeks the labia nearly cover the clitoris, and at 40-plus weeks the labia majora completely cover the clitoris.
The nurse completes the assessment by observation. **Male genitals** are evaluated for size of the scrotal sac, presence of rugae, and descent of the testes. The nurse observes the size of the scrotal sac and the presence or absence of rugae. The scrotal sac can be gently palpated to determine descent of the testes.

Neuromuscular characteristics

a. **Resting posture** should be assessed as the baby lies undisturbed on a flat surface such as his or her bed.

b. **Square window (wrist)** is elicited by flexing the baby's hand toward the ventral forearm. The angle formed at the wrist is measured (by estimation and matching it against the angles on the scoring tool) (see Figure 5–5).

c. **Arm recoil** is a test of flexion development. It is best evaluated after the first hour of life when the baby has had time to recover from the stress of birth. To assess, place the newborn in a supine position (lying on his/her back), completely flex both elbows (by holding the newborn's hands and placing the hands up against the forearms),

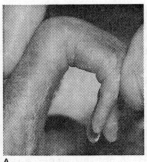

A

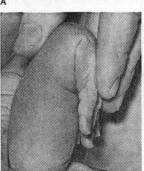

C

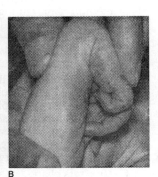

B

Figure 5–5   Square window sign. A, This angle is 90° and suggests an immature newborn of 28 to 32 weeks' gestation. B, A 30° angle is commonly found from 38 to 40 weeks' gestation. C, A 0° angle occurs from 40 to 42 weeks. (From Dubowitz L, Dubowitz V: Gestational Age of the Newborn. Menlo Park: CA, Addison-Wesley Nursing, 1977.)

hold them in this position for about five seconds, and then release them. On release, the elbows of a full-term newborn form an angle of less than 90° and rapidly recoil back to flexed position. The arms of a preterm have slower recoil time and form greater than a 90° angle.

d. **Popliteal angle** is determined with the newborn supine and flat. The thigh is flexed on the abdomen/chest, and the nurse places the index finger of the other hand behind the newborn's ankle to extend the lower leg until resistance is met. The angle formed is then measured. Results vary from no resistance in the very immature infant to an 80° angle in the term infant.

e. **Scarf sign** is elicited by placing the neonate supine and drawing an arm across the chest toward the infant's opposite shoulder. The arm is pulled until resistance is met. (The newborn needs to remain lying on his/her back. The location of the elbow is then noted in relation to the midline of the chest) (see Figure 5–6).

f. **Heel to ear** is performed by placing the baby in a supine position and, while stabilizing the hip on the bed, gently drawing the foot toward the ear on the same side until resistance is felt. Both the popliteal angle and the proximity of the foot to the ear are assessed. In a very preterm newborn, the leg will remain straight and the foot will go to the ear or beyond. If the newborn was in a breech presentation, this assessment should be delayed until the legs are positioned more normally.

Scoring All individual scores are added and the total number is compared to the score on the Estimation of Gestational Age by Maturity Rating tool. A score of 35 equals 38 weeks, a score of 37 equals 39 weeks, and a score of 40 equals 40 weeks.

The estimated gestational age is plotted on a tool that classifies newborns by birth weight and gestational age (see Figure 5–7). Most newborns are appropriate for gestational age (AGA). A baby that is large for gestational age (LGA) or small for gestational age (SGA) may require additional assessment and intervention (for further discussion see Chapter 6).

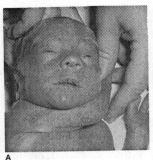
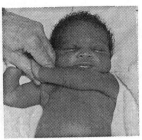
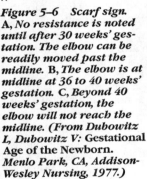
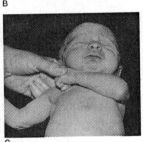

Figure 5–6 Scarf sign. A, No resistance is noted until after 30 weeks' gestation. The elbow can be readily moved past the midline. B, The elbow is at midline at 36 to 40 weeks' gestation. C, Beyond 40 weeks' gestation, the elbow will not reach the midline. (From Dubowitz L, Dubowitz V: Gestational Age of the Newborn. Menlo Park, CA, Addison-Wesley Nursing, 1977.)

4. Administer erythromycin (Ilotycin) ointment (or silver nitrate drops) into the newborn's eyes. This is a legally required prophylactic eye treatment for *Neisseria gonorrhoea,* which may have infected the newborn during the birth process. Ilotycin has the advantage of being useful for both gonorrhea and *Chlamydia;* it is also less irritating to the newborn's eyes, which results in decreased incidence of swelling and discharge.

5. Administer prophylactic dose of vitamin K. The vitamin K is given to prevent hemorrhage, which can occur because of low prothrombin levels in the first few days of life (see Figure 5–8 for injection sites).

6. Assess glucose level. A drop of blood is obtained by heel stick and blood glucose is determined (see Figure 5–9). The glucose strip should read > 45 mg/dL; a value < 45 mg/dL needs to be followed up by

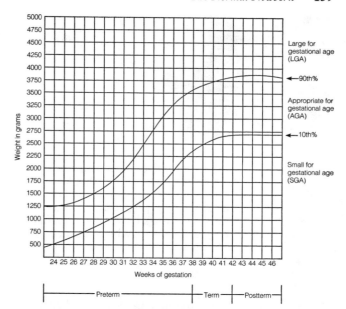

Figure 5–7   Classification of newborns by birth weight and gestational age. The newborn's birth weight and gestational age are plotted on the graph. The newborn is then classified as large for gestational age (LGA), appropriate for gestational age (AGA), or small for gestational age (SGA). For example, a baby of 38 weeks' gestation who weighs 2875 gm is considered AGA. (From Battaglia FC, Lubchenco LO: A practical classification of newborn infants by weight and gestational age. J Pediatr *1967; 71:161.)*

Figure 5–8   Newborn injection sites. The middle third of the vastus lateralis muscle is the preferred site for intramuscular injection in the newborn.

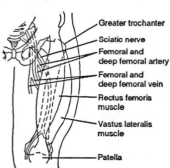

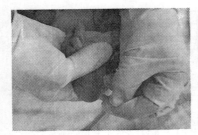

Figure 5–9 Blood is obtained by a heel stick for a glucose (Chemstrip) test.

drawing a central blood sample (drawn from a vein in the hand or antecubital space) for further laboratory evaluation. Treatment is begun if needed (see Chapter 6 for discussion of hypoglycemia). **Be alert for:** Hypoglycemia in high-risk babies such as SGA, infant of diabetic mother (IDM), AGA preterm, and any newborn that was stressed during labor and at birth. Outward signs of hypoglycemia may include lethargy, jitteriness, poor feeding, vomiting, pallor, apnea, irregular respirations, and/or tremors.

7. Maintain temperature through use of a controlled radiant warmer. A probe is placed on the newborn's abdomen just under the ribs or over the area of the liver. The probe indicates the newborn's temperature, and the radiant heater responds by becoming warmer or cooler. **Be alert for:** Newborns at risk for hypothermia (temperature < 97.7F), including preterms, SGA, and any baby that was stressed at birth.

   If the newborn's temperature is 97.7F or below (axillary or skin probe temperature), rewarming is needed. The baby is placed under a radiant warmer, undressed so that the skin can be warmed, and the warmer set for 98.6F. When the skin probe indicates that the desired temperature has been reached, recheck axillary temperature. The baby may be removed from the warmer; however, axillary temperature should be rechecked about every 30 minutes for an hour or so to make sure the baby is maintaining a normal temperature.

   Successful transition to extrauterine existence is documented by stabilization of vital signs and establishment of awake/sleep cycles and feeding, stooling, and voiding patterns.

POST-TRANSITIONAL NURSING CARE

Overview

Once the newborn has passed through the transitional period, he/she is transferred to a normal newborn area. Normal newborn care usually includes assessment of vital signs (axillary temperature, apical pulse, and respirations) every four hours, a physical assessment every eight hours, application of a drying agent to the umbilical stump every eight hours, feeding every three to four hours, diapering as needed, and weighing once every 24 hours.

Physical Assessment

It is usually easier to proceed from head to toe; however, you need to assess axillary temperature, apical pulse, and respirations while the baby is quiet. Completing the assessment in the mother's room provides a wonderful opportunity for teaching, sharing, and role modeling for first-time mothers.

1. **Head.** Palpate and observe fontanelles. The anterior fontanelle is the largest and is diamond shaped. The posterior fontanelle is triangular in shape. The sagittal suture (located on the top of the head, from front to back) is smooth and without ridges.
   Common variations: bulging of fontanelle (increased intracranial pressure), depressed fontanelle (dehydration), overriding of sagittal suture (molding), caput succedaneum (edema in tissues from trauma), cephalhematoma (bleeding into the periosteal space).
   Be alert for: Premature closing of both anterior and posterior sutures and overriding of sutures (craniosynostosis) requires further assessment.

2. **Eyes.** Inspect eyes and lids. Eyes should be clear, without drainage, and no swelling of eyelids. Subconjunctival hemorrhage may be present.
   Common variations: swelling of eyelid (birth trauma, reaction to eye prophylaxis).
   Be alert for: Purulent drainage is an indication for further assessment and treatment.

3. **Ears.** Inspect outer ear. A full-term baby has incurving of the top two-thirds of the pinna. The top of the

ear should be above an imaginary line drawn from the inner canthus to the outer canthus of the eye and extended around toward the ear. Rotation of the ear should be in the midline, and not tipped forward or backward.

Be alert for: Low-set ears may be associated with a variety of congenital problems.

4. **Nose.** Inspect. Nares should be clear and without mucus. (Remember, newborn is an obligatory nose breather, so a stuffy nose has much greater implications for a newborn baby.)

Common variations: none.

Be alert for: Assess for presence of nasal flaring. If present, assess respiratory rate, retractions and grunting, and skin color. A pulse-oximeter determination may provide further information (reading should be above 90%).

5. **Mouth.** Inspect inside of mouth and palpate hard palate. Hard and soft palate should be intact (may visualize while the baby is crying or may palpate with a gloved finger). (An opening indicates cleft palate.) Inspect gums for supernumerary teeth (these teeth usually do not cause a problem but may loosen and fall out unexpectedly).

Common variations: supernumerary teeth and Epstein's pearls.

Be alert for: An opening in the palate (cleft palate) needs to be evaluated quickly. Presence of white patches on the mucous membranes that appear as milk deposits but cannot be wiped away with a 4×4 may indicate thrush *(Candida)*. Excessive mucus may be associated with atresia.

6. **Chest.** Inspect. Chest should be symmetric. Breasts may be flat or slightly enlarged because of the effects of maternal estrogen (this may last about one week). Count respiratory rate over one minute (uncover baby and look at movement of chest or abdomen).

Common variations: supernumerary nipple.

Be alert for: If retractions (intercostal or sternal) are present, assess respiratory rate and determine baby's need for oxygen.

7. **Heart.** Auscultate. Apical pulse ranges from 120 to 160 bpm. May be as low as 100 with sleep. Palpate brachial, radial, femoral, and pedal pulses.
Common variations: A transitory murmur may be heard for the first few hours of life.
Be alert for: Bradycardia (< 100 bpm) or tachycardia (> 160 bpm) need further evaluation.

8. **Abdomen.** Inspect, auscultate, palpate. Abdomen should be flat (without distention), and bowel sounds should be heard in all quadrants. Umbilical stump should be drying and have no redness, discharge, or bleeding.
Common variations: none.
Be alert for: Bleeding and/or purulent drainage from cord require further assessment and treatment.

9. **Genitals.** Inspect. Genitals should be clearly differentiated. Both testes should be palpable in scrotum.
Common variations: pseudomenstruation (small amount vaginal bleeding) in female infants due to maternal estrogen exposure. Clear mucus from the vagina, vaginal skin tag.
Be alert for: Urinary meatus on the underside of the penis (hypospadias).

10. **Back.** Inspect. Back should be smooth with no tufts of hair present over the lower back.
Common variations: mongolian spot over lower back.

11. **Hips.** Inspect and perform Ortolani maneuver to detect subluxation or congenital dislocation of hips. Legs should be of equal length, skin folds on both right and left posterior thighs should be symmetric (see Figure 5–10). To do Ortolani maneuver, place newborn on her/his back. Place the palm of your right hand on the newborn's left knee and extend your index and middle finger toward the hip. Your fingertips should be on the top of the greater trochanter. Place your left hand in the same manner. Put downward pressure on the knees and rotate the knees outward. Feel for a "click" under your fingertips. If a click is felt, notify baby's care provider. The baby will most likely be triple diapered to keep the hip abducted.

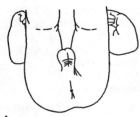

A

Figure 5–10
A, *Congenital dislocated right hip in a young infant as seen on gross inspection.*
B, *Barlow (dislocation) test. Baby's thigh is grasped as above and adducted with gentle downward pressure. Dislocation is palpable as femoral head slips out of acetabulum.*
C, *Ortolani's maneuver puts downward pressure on the hip and then inward rotation. If the hip is dislocated, this pressure will force the femoral head over the acetabular rim with a noticeable "clunk." (Smith DW:* Recognizable Patterns of Human Deformation. *Philadelphia: Saunders, 1981.)*

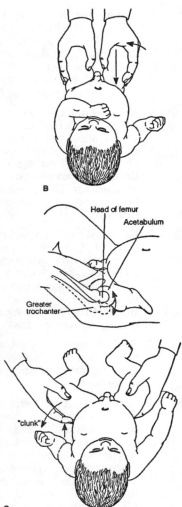

B

C

12. **Extremities.** Inspect. All extremities should be symmetric and move equally. Count digits on hands and feet; inspect palmar creases. Note any webbing (syndactyly).
    Common variations: none.

Be alert for: Asymmetric movement or no movement of an extremity needs to be reported and assessed further.

13. **Skin color.** Inspect. Skin color appropriate for ethnic grouping. Any evidence of acrocyanosis usually should have abated. Observe closely for signs of jaundice. Jaundice is first detectable on the face, the mucous membranes of the mouth, and the sclera. It is evaluated by blanching the tip of the nose or the forehead. If jaundice is present, the area will appear yellowish immediately after blanching. Laboratory testing will verify the total bilirubin level.

    Common variations: Milia may be present over the nose. A variety of markings may be present on the skin (see Table 5–4).

    Be alert for: Cyanosis requires immediate reassessment and treatment. Jaundice requires additional assessment, evaluation, and then treatment as needed. Pallor may be associated with anemia, and ruddiness may indicate an elevated hematocrit (> 65%).

    Newborns with levels above 10–11 mg/dL may be placed under phototherapy. A newborn under

Table 5–4   Birthmarks

Type	Characteristics	Parent Teaching
Telangiectatic nevi (stork bites)	Pale pink or red flat dilated capillaries over eyelids, nose, and nape of neck	Seen more with crying Blanch easily, fade during infancy, gone by 2 years of age
Mongolian spots	Bluish-black macular areas over dorsal area and buttocks	Common in dark-skinned races Gradually fade in 1st–2nd year of life
Nevus flammeus (port-wine stain)	Nonelevated, sharply outlined, red-purple dense area of capillaries, primarily on face In black infants appears jet black	Doesn't fade with time nor blanch as a rule. Can cover with opaque cosmetic cream. Suggestive of Sturge-Weber syndrome (involving 5th cranial nerve)

phototherapy needs to be blindfolded (to protect eyes from the lights), undressed (to allow ultraviolet light to shine on skin), rotated every 30–60 minutes (for even exposure), fed adequate amounts of breast milk and/or water (to stimulate intestinal movement of absorbed bilirubin), and soothed frequently (being undressed and unwrapped can make the baby feel uncomfortable).

14. **Elimination.** Note newborn record. Newborn should void and stool within 24 hours after birth. After that, most babies have six to eight wet diapers a day and may stool at least once a day. Breastfed babies tend to have more frequent stools.
    Common variations: none.
    Be alert for: If baby does not void within 24 hours, assess amount of fluid taken in, assess urethral opening. If no stool, assess abdomen for distention and bowel sounds. In some settings, a rectal thermometer coated with a lubricant is inserted (about 1/2 inch) into the rectum to stimulate the stool. Check on agency policy before attempting. Diarrhea stools can be very serious for the newborn. Observe stool characteristics closely, and test the stool for occult blood (Hematest) and sugar loss (Clinitest or other glucose testing).

15. **Behavioral.** Observe. Baby quiets to soothing, cuddling, or wrapping. Moves through all sleep-awake states.
    Common variations: none.
    Be alert for: Excessive crying, fretfulness, and inability to quiet self may be associated with drug withdrawal in the neonate.

    Tip: Completing the assessment in the mother's room provides a wonderful opportunity for teaching, sharing, and role modeling for first-time mothers.

Assessment of Reflexes

At some point during the time you spend with this newborn, assess normal newborn reflexes.

1. **Moro.** Elicited by startling the newborn with a loud noise, or sudden movement. Newborn straightens

arms and hands out while flexing knees. The arms then return to the chest as in an embrace. The fingers spread, forming a C, and the infant may cry.

2. **Grasp.** Elicited by stimulating the newborn's palm with a finger or object. The newborn grasps and holds the object or finger firmly enough to be lifted momentarily from the crib.

3. **Rooting.** Elicited when the side of the newborn's mouth or cheek is touched. In response, the newborn turns toward that side and opens the lips to suck.

Documenting Assessment Findings and Care

Assessment findings may be recorded on computer charting systems, neonatal flow sheets, or in narrative notes. A narrative note might be recorded as follows:

> Anterior fontanelle soft and flat, posterior fontanelle palpated closed at this time, some molding present with overriding of sagittal suture, caput succedaneum over posterior aspect of head. Eyes clear and without discharge or swelling. Nares clear without flaring or discharge. Mouth clear, and palate palpated intact. Chest movements symmetrical without retractions, apical pulse 134, regular, and no murmurs auscultated. Abdomen soft and nondistended. Baby has had a meconium and transitional stool, bowel sounds × 4. Umbilical stump drying and is without redness or discharge. Alcohol applied. No redness or discharge noted on genitalia. Perineal area cleansed and A and D ointment applied. Back clear. Moves all extremities equally. No hip click. Palmar creases normal. Skin color appropriate to ethnic group and without cyanosis. Soothes with cuddling and rocking. M.Chin, RNC

Additional Aspects of Daily Care

1. **Suctioning.** Achieved by compressing the bulb syringe, inserting it into the side of the mouth, and then releasing the bulb. The bulb should be withdrawn, the contents expelled onto a paper towel or cloth. The bulb is then recompressed and placed back into the mouth if needed. It is best to have the bulb available at all times for the newborn. It is important to teach the parents the use of the bulb at

their first contact with the baby. Some parents are frightened of the bulb, and it helps for them to actually hold it and compress it. When choking occurs, the baby may be picked up, held with her/his head slightly down and the mouth to the side to facilitate the drainage of mucus. It can be frightening to deal with a choking baby.

2. **Positioning.** Place the baby on his/her right side following feedings with a rolled blanket at the back to hold him/her in this position. The baby can be placed on the tummy after the cord (and circumcision if done) heals. A newborn should never be placed on her/his back because of the risk of choking.

3. **Wrapping.** The newborn seems to be comforted by being wrapped snugly in blankets (see Figure 5–11).

4. **Holding.** To pick up the newborn, take hold of the feet with one hand, and slide the other hand up under the baby until you reach the back of the shoulders and neck. The baby can now be picked up and placed up over your shoulder, or cradled in the crook of your arm. (Sometimes it is easier to place the baby against your shoulder first, get settled, and then change the baby to the crook of your arm. If you are right handed, you will tend to be most comfortable cradling the baby in your left arm. Remember to teach new parents this technique.) The baby may also be held in a football hold.

5. **Circumcision care.** Some parents choose to have their male newborn circumcised. Prior to the pro-

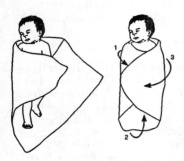

Figure 5–11   Steps used for wrapping a baby.

cedure, the parents need to validate that they understand the procedure and sign an informed consent. After the circumcision, the penis needs to be assessed for bleeding. If a Gomco clamp is used, A and D ointment is applied at each diaper change to provide protection to the skin and keep the penis from sticking to the diaper. If a Plastibell is used, the remaining plastic ring protects the penis. Other than cleansing by letting warm water softly rinse over the penis to clear away urine, no other care is required. The Plastibell usually falls off by itself in about three to four days. If it is still in place in seven days, the parents need to contact their care provider.

Comfort measures immediately after the circumcision may include wrapping the baby in soft blankets and rocking, walking with the baby, using a pacifier, feeding after initial crying has abated, singing, gently rubbing the back, talking to the baby, and using therapeutic touch (use short, light, feathery strokes for a short period of time).

6. **Testing for phenylketonuria (PKU).** Prior to the newborn's discharge, blood needs to be obtained by heel stick for PKU testing. A second test will be done in 7–14 days, and it is important to stress the need for the second test with the parents. It is usually done on an outpatient basis.

7. In many settings, the pediatrician orders the first Heptovax injection to be given prior to discharge.

Parent Education

Provide information as needed on the following topics:

1. **Axillary temperature.** To use a glass thermometer, you must first shake the mercury down below the numbers and then place the thermometer in the baby's right or left axilla. The thermometer needs to be in contact with skin on all sides (see Figure 5–12). Hold the thermometer in place for three minutes. It is important to keep your hand on the thermometer at all times to ensure correct placement and prevent an accident. After reading the temperature, cleanse the thermometer by rinsing in cool water and wiping with a soft towel. Review normal range

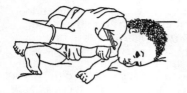

Figure 5–12 The axillary temperature should be taken for three minutes. The newborn's arm should be tightly but gently pressed against the thermometer and the newborn's side.

of temperature (axillary: 97.8 to 99F). **Teaching Tip:** Make a thermometer out of poster board. The mercury can be simulated with aluminum foil. Or, warm a thermometer between your fingers (if this is the first time you have taught the class it probably won't work because your fingers will be very cold!). You may find it helpful to tell the parents what the temperature is before passing the thermometer around, as many parents may feel uncomfortable telling you they cannot read a thermometer. Tell parents to let you know at the end of class if they would like any assistance or a review.

2. **Bathing the newborn.** Collect supplies (see Table 5–5). For the first few baths, schedule uninterrupted time if at all possible. Wash baby's face using a washcloth that has been moistened in warm water but does not contain soap. The eyes are done first (while the washcloth is the most clean). Using a corner of the washcloth around your finger, wipe the right eye from the inner canthus to the outer can-

---

Table 5–5   Bath Time Supplies

A plastic tub	Vitamin A and D ointment (for dry skin)
Two bath towels or baby blankets	70% isopropyl alcohol
Two washcloths	Cotton balls or Q-tips™ for alcohol application
Mild soap (unperfumed is best because it is not as drying to the baby's skin)	

---

thus, in one stroke. If another swipe is needed, use another corner of the washcloth. The left eye is washed in the same manner. Then the face is washed, as well as under the chin, and then dried. You may choose to wash the baby's hair at this point or at the end of the bath. (Those most interested in organization and saving steps would say to shampoo the hair now; others would say it needs to be done at the end of the bath to better maintain the newborn's temperature.) The chest and abdomen are then washed, rinsed, and dried. You can either use your hands or a washcloth. Umbilical care is completed by cleansing around the umbilical stump with a cotton ball that has a small amount of alcohol applied. Be sure not to oversaturate the cotton ball (it is too wet if alcohol drips from it). The diaper is removed. If bathing a male baby, be sure to keep a diaper or rag at hand in case the baby urinates (a male infant is able to spray the urine on you). Carefully and gently clean from the area of the symphysis (pubic bone) down toward the anus. Use a separate portion of the washcloth for each motion. The baby's back and buttocks may be washed, rinsed, and dried. If the hair has not yet been washed, carefully wrap the baby in a dry blanket. Use a football hold to support the baby safely and yet have one hand free for shampooing. Wet the baby's hair and apply a mild shampoo. Lather, rinse thoroughly, and dry. You may want to make a hood over the baby's wet hair until the baby is completely dressed and rewarmed after the bath. Brushing the baby's hair stimulates the scalp and also removes dead skin cells and prevents cradle cap.

3. **Nails.** The nails may be trimmed with special baby-sized cuticle/nail scissors. Clippers may be too large to allow you to see the baby's nails.

4. **Diapering with reusable cloth diapers.** Many diaper-folding methods are available, as well as diaper wraps that allow the diaper to be placed inside a Velcro™-fastened wrapper (see Figure 5–13).

5. **Diapering with single-use paper diapers.** The baby is placed on the diaper, the front is pulled up toward the navel, and the sides are brought forward

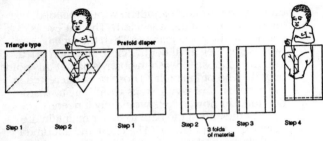

Figure 5–13 Two methods of using cloth diapers.

and attached by a sticky tab to the front of the diaper. Care needs to be followed to fold the diaper below the level of the umbilicus for the first seven to ten days. In addition, soiled diapers should not be left in open waste containers.

6. **Highlights of parent teaching for newborn care.**

Cord care	Complete cord care two to four times/day. Cord falls off in seven to ten days.
Perineal care	Wash and dry diaper area with each diaper change.
Circumcision care	If Gomco clamp was used, apply A and D ointment with each diaper change. If Plastibell was used, do NOT apply ointment. Plastibell falls off in three to four days. Contact care provider if it has not fallen off in seven days. Cleanse penis by letting warm water flow over penis after each voiding. Do NOT attempt to remove whitish area on skin.
Bath	Give sponge baths until cord has fallen off and area healed (about 10–14 days). Then tub bath may be given.

	Bathe every other day (or every third day) in dry climates. Those in warm, humid climates may bathe baby every day.
Axillary temperature	Shake mercury down below numbers. Leave in place at least three minutes, positioned so skin contacts the thermometer on all sides. Normal findings are 97.8F to 99F.
When to call	Water-loss stools (small amount of stool surrounded by a ring of water in the diaper) Axillary temperature of > 101F or < 97.6F Any color change involving pallor or cyanosis Refusing two feedings in a row Vomiting, especially projectile Failure to have at least six wet diapers each day Crying that persists for two to three hours and the baby cannot be soothed Lethargy or listlessness

CHAPTER 6

The At-Risk Newborn

HYPOGLYCEMIA

Overview

Hypoglycemia is a condition of abnormally low levels of serum glucose. It can be defined as a blood glucose level below 40 mg/dL after birth for all newborns; or a glucose oxidase reagent strip reading below 45 mg/dL when corroborated by a blood glucose test. In clinical practice, an infant with a blood glucose level less than 45 mg/dL requires intervention. Hypoglycemia can be asymptomatic or symptomatic. Presentation of symptoms and blood glucose levels vary greatly with each baby. Symptoms usually occur at < 45 mg/dL and appear between 24 and 72 hours after birth or within 6 hours after birth in severely stressed infants. A glucose level of 45 mg/dL or more by 72 hours of age is the goal regardless of weight, gestational age, or other predisposing factors. Clinical manifestations vary greatly but can include tremors or jittery movements, irritability, lethargy or hypotonia, irregular respirations, apnea, cyanosis, refusal to suck, high-pitched or weak cry, hypothermia, diaphoresis, or neonatal seizure activity. When left untreated, hypoglycemia can cause cerebral damage and mental retardation.

Medical Management

Drug therapy. Initially, 5% to 10% glucose is given with a followup blood glucose test within 30–60 minutes after feeding. If the baby can't take oral glucose, a 5%–10% glucose intravenous infusion is ordered at a rate which gives 6–8 mg/kg/min of glucose (@90–100 mL/kg/day). For symptomatic acute hypoglycemia a bolus dose of

D10W IV at rate of 1–2 mL/kg is given followed by 10% glucose infusion. Alternative treatment may be: hydrocortisone 5 mg/kg p.o. q12hrs after 6–12 hours of glucose treatment, or glucagon 0.3 mg/kg IM only as an emergency treatment. Insulin infusion drip may be preferred to glucagon administration.

Critical Nursing Assessments

1. Assess newborn and record for any risk factors.
   Be alert for: Special gestational newborns, such as premature, small for gestational age (SGA), and infant of diabetic mother (IDM) infants, and newborns with problems of asphyxia, cold stress, sepsis, or polycythemia are particularly at risk. Also maternal epidural anesthesia can alter maternal-fetal glucose homeostasis.

2. Assess dextrostix or blood glucose chemstrip on all newborns within one to two hours of birth (see Procedure: Glucose Chemstrip Test Using Accu-Check II Machine). In high-risk infants, routine screening should be carried out 2, 4, 6, 12, 24, and 48 hours of age or whenever any of the clinical manifestations appear and then until stable.

3. Assess all newborns for symptoms of hypoglycemia.

Sample Nursing Diagnoses

- Pain related to multiple heel sticks for glucose monitoring.
- Altered nutrition: less than body requirements related to increased glucose use secondary to physiologic stresses.
- Ineffective family coping related to fear over infant's condition.

Critical Nursing Interventions

1. Based on agency glucose testing protocol, provide early feedings of breastmilk or 5% glucose for infants at risk for hypoglycemia.

2. Obtain chemstrip blood glucose per agency protocol. If < 45 mg/dL, obtain STAT blood glucose

per venous stick by lab. Then provide oral glucose water (about 1 oz) to infant. Recheck chemstrip in one hour.

Note: If initial chemstrip is < 20 mg/dL, obtain STAT blood glucose and prepare to start IV glucose therapy.

3. Monitor all babies for signs and symptoms of hypoglycemia.

4. Monitor infants with low chemstrips who have been given oral glucose water for rebound hypoglycemia in approximately three to four hours.

5. If IV therapy is ordered by the physician or indicated by your agency protocol:

   a. Start 10% dextrose and water IV on infusion pump on infants at risk for hypoglycemia or give bolus for symptomatic infants then continue glucose infusion as ordered.

   b. Administer infusion in peripheral vein of upper extremity to avoid lower extremity varicosities and potential tissue necrosis if IV infiltrates.

   c. Obtain glucose levels using chemstrip or dextrostix hourly during therapy until condition stabilizes. Obtain blood glucose levels q4–8hrs minimum.

6. Calculate glucose intake from all sources (IV and oral).

7. Monitor titration of IV glucose during transition to oral glucose.

8. Provide comfort measures to ensure rest, and maintain the optimal thermal environment specific for each newborn to reduce activity and glucose consumption.

9. Assist parents to identify feelings and concerns about baby's condition. Encourage and allow for maximum contact between parents and their baby.

10. Review the following critical aspects of the care you have provided:

    • Did I identify the baby's risk for hypoglycemia early in its care?

- Have I been alert for the early signs of hypoglycemia?
- Have I monitored the blood glucose levels carefully and instituted care per agency protocol promptly?

Sample Nurse's Charting

6:25 AM T 97.7F, P 150, R 35 & periodic. Ant. fontanelle soft & flat. Breath sounds equal bilaterally, slight substernal retractions. Abdomen soft and nondistended. Hypoactive bowel sounds. Fine tremors of arms and hands.

Essential Precautions in Practice

During Care of At-Risk Newborns

Examples of times when disposable gloves should be worn include the following:

- Handling baby prior to first bath, even when all blood and amniotic fluid has been removed
- Suctioning oral and nasal secretions
- During resuscitation, with use of bag and mask ventilation
- Administering vitamin K injection, eye prophylaxis, and cord care
- Carrying out routine heel stick blood work (eg, glucose, hematocrit)
- Inserting umbilical catheter lines—umbilical artery (UAC) and umbilical vein (UVC)—and any other invasive lines
- Flushing and blood drawing from umbilical catheter lines (UAC, UVC)

All invasive procedures require sterile gloves and should be carried out over thoroughly cleansed areas of skin. At times goggles and protective gowns or aprons may be required.

REMEMBER to wash your hands prior to putting the disposable gloves on and AGAIN immediately after you remove the gloves. For further information consult OSHA and CDC guidelines.

Chemstrip 38 mg/dL. Poor suck, took 25 mL of G/W with difficulty. Lab blood glucose pending. Dr. Rich notified of glucose level. M. Chin, RN.

Evaluation

Anticipated outcomes of nursing care include:

- Newborn's glucose level is stable at > 45 mg/dL, and the baby is symptom free.
- Newborn is free from further complications.

COLD STRESS

Overview

Cold stress occurs when babies are placed in an environment colder than their neutral thermal environment. When babies become chilled, they increase their oxygen consumption and use of glucose for physiologic processes. The complications that occur because of this alteration in metabolic processes are respiratory distress, respiratory and metabolic acidosis, hypoglycemia, and jaundice. Premature, SGA, hypoxic, hypoglycemic, and central nervous system (CNS) depressed newborns are at higher risk for becoming hypothermic and suffer the consequences.

Medical Management

Initially, medical management is directed to prevention and then to the management required by the specific complication.

Critical Nursing Assessments

1. Assess newborn temperature, using either axillary or skin probe method.
   Be alert for: A drop in skin temperature (it drops before core temperature), which may be an early indicator of cold stress. **Tip:** Axillary temperature can be misleading because of the nearness to brown fat, which can increase heat production.

2. Assess for signs of hypothermia: Shallow, irregular respirations, retractions, diminished reflexes, bradycardia, oliguria, lethargy, and temperature < 97.8F.

3. Assess for complications such as hyperbilirubinemia, hypoglycemia (blood glucose < 45 mg/dL), and respiratory distress.

Sample Nursing Diagnoses

- Hypothermia related to exposure to cold environment, trauma, illness, or inability to shiver.
- Ineffective thermoregulation related to immaturity.
- Knowledge deficit related to lack of information about maintenance of neutral thermal environment.

Critical Nursing Interventions

1. Institute measures to prevent heat loss due to radiation, evaporation, convection, and conduction. Measures include: Dry off baby immediately and remove wet linen after birth; place baby on pre-warmed bed under radiant heat source for all care and procedures, cover scales before weighing, warm stethoscope bell prior to auscultation; keep beds away from drafts and air vents, use warmed humidified oxygen, keep baby wrapped when not skin to skin, or cover head with stockinette hat or place under radiant heat source with temperature probe in place; turn up thermostat in birthing area prior to birth; do not place warmer bed near windows or outside walls.

2. If chilled: Rewarm slowly to prevent apnea (see Procedure 17: Temperature Stabilization of the Newborn).

3. Monitor blood glucose levels for signs of hypoglycemia and arterial blood gases for signs of respiratory distress.

4. Carry out care needed by newborns placed under phototherapy to maintain stable temperature. (See the section on jaundice in this chapter.)

5. Instruct parents about causes of temperature fluctuation, infant's current status, heat-conservation methods, and temperature-stabilization methods.

6. Review the following critical aspects of the care you have provided:

- Have I provided for sufficient warmth during all procedures and care activities? During baths? During IV starts or blood work?
- Have I been alert for any signs of hypoglycemia, hyperbilirubinemia, or respiratory distress?

Evaluation

Anticipated outcomes of nursing care include:

- Baby is maintained in a neutral thermal environment.
- Parents understand the importance of preventing heat loss and methods to prevent complications of hypothermia.

RESPIRATORY DISTRESS SYNDROME

Overview

Respiratory distress syndrome (RDS) is a condition that affects approximately 40,000 to 50,000 infants a year in the United States. The main factors associated with the development of RDS are primarily prematurity and any factor resulting in a deficiency of functioning surfactant, eg, a diabetic mother or hypoxia. Clinical manifestations may present at birth or within a few hours after birth. The general clinical manifestations are tachypnea, expiratory grunting, nasal flaring on inspiration, and subcostal/intercostal retractions. Other clinical manifestations include pallor and cyanosis, apnea, labored breathing, increasing need for oxygen, and hypotonus. The x-ray shows diffuse reticulogranular density bilaterally with portions of the air-filled tracheobronchial tree (air bronchogram) outlined by the opaque lungs. RDS usually resolves over 4–7 days unless surfactant replacement therapy has been used. A frequent complication is patent ductus arteriosus.

Medical Management

Supportive management involves oxygen administration, ventilation therapy, blood gas studies to monitor oxygen and carbon dioxide levels, transcutaneous or pulse oximeter methods, and correction of acid-base imbalance. Ventilatory therapy is aimed at preventing hypoventilation and hypoxia. The degree of ventilatory support needed ranges from increasing oxygen concentration to the use of continuous positive airway pressure (CPAP) to intubation and full mechanical ventilation. Surfactant-replacement therapy, both artificial surfactant (Exosurf) and modified natural surfactant (Survanta), has been shown to improve oxygenation rapidly and decrease the need for ventilatory support. Surfactant-replacement therapy must be administered by specially trained personnel.

Critical Nursing Assessment

1. Assess newborn and record any risk factors.
   Be alert for: Special gestational newborns such as premature infants and any infant suspected of hypoxia in utero or soon after birth.

2. Assess newborn's respiratory effort. Note chest wall movement and respiratory effort (grunting, nasal flaring, retractions), color (cyanosis, pallor, duskiness) of skin and mucous membranes, auscultation of lung for bilateral air entry.
   Tip: At about 48–72 hrs (if no surfactant-replacement therapy is given), when the alveoli begin to open up, watch the chest movement carefully, because the infant is at greatest risk for pneumothorax at that time.

3. Assess need for increased oxygen and assisted ventilation measures.
   Note: Normal PaO_2: 50–70 mm Hg, $PaCO_2$: 35–45 mm Hg, and pH 7.35–7.45. Monitor blood pressure (average for term infant, 74/47; preterm infant, 64/39).

4. Assess I&O and electrolytes. Increased labored breathing (work of breathing) causes an increase in insensible water losses.
   Tip: As the lungs open up, there is usually an increase in voiding because more fluid moves into the bloodstream to be excreted by the kidneys.

5. Assess for signs of infection: temperature instability, lethargy, poor feeding, hypotonia.

Sample Nursing Diagnoses

- Impaired gas exchange related to inadequate lung surfactant.
- Altered nutrition: less than body requirements related to increased metabolic needs of stressed infant.
- Risk for infection related to invasive procedures.
- Ineffective thermoregulation related to increased respiratory effort secondary to RDS.

Critical Nursing Interventions

1. Administer warmed, humidified oxygen by designated route: oxygen hood, continuous positive airway pressure (CPAP), and intubation (Figure 6–1).

2. Alter oxygen concentrations by 5%–10% increments or per order to maintain adequate PaO_2 levels. Obtain blood gas levels after any significant change in oxygen concentration.

3. Obtain arterial blood gases per order. Maintain stable environment prior to blood gas studies (do not suction, change oxygen levels or ventilator settings, or disturb baby).

4. Suction as necessary. Secretions are sparse until 2nd–3rd day when the lungs start opening up. Watch transcutaneous oxygen monitor or pulse oximeter for desatuaration during procedure.

5. Check and calibrate all monitoring and measuring devices every 8 hours.

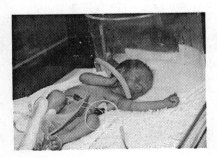

Figure 6–1
Infant in oxygen hood.

6. Maintain adequate I&O. Maintain patency of IVs.

7. Maintain a neutral thermal enviroment. Temperature instability increases oxygen consumption and metabolic acidosis.

8. Administer medications per order: antibiotics, diuretics, sedatives, and analgesics. Fentanyl as well as morphine are used for their analgesic and sedative effects. The use of pancuronium (Pavulon) for muscle relaxation is controversial.

9. Careful hand washing, use of gloves during procedures, and attention to infection control are essential.

10. Provide time to answer parents' questions about the baby's status and the equipment used, and to give emotional support. Explain developmental supportive care to the parents.

11. Record and report all clinical observations.

Evaluation

Anticipated outcomes of nursing care include:

- The risk of RDS is promptly identified, and early intervention is initiated.
- The newborn is free of respiratory distress and metabolic alterations.
- The parents verbalize their concerns about their baby's health problem/survival and understand the rationale behind management of their newborn.

SPECIAL NEWBORNS AND THEIR ASSOCIATED CLINICAL PROBLEMS

Classification	Physical Characteristics	Clinical Problems
Small for gestational age (SGA)	Large-appearing head in proportion to chest and abdomen Loose, dry skin	1. **Perinatal asphyxia.** Chronic hypoxia in utero leaves little reserve to withstand the demands of labor and birth. Thus,

Classification	Physical Characteristics	Clinical Problems
Small for gestational age (SGA) *(continued)*	Scarcity of subcutaneous fat, with emaciated appearance	intrauterine asphyxia occurs with its potential systemic problems.
	Long, thin appearance	2. **Aspiration syndromes.** Gasping secondary to in utero hypoxia can cause aspiration of amniotic fluid into the lower airways, or can lead to relaxation of the anal sphincter with passage of meconium. This results in meconium aspiration with first breaths after birth.
	Sunken abdomen	
	Sparse scalp hair	
	Anterior fontanelle may be depressed	
	May have vigorous cry and appears alert	
	Birth weight below tenth percentile	3. **Heat loss.** Decreased ability to conserve heat results from diminished subcutaneous fat (used for survival in utero), depletion of brown fat in utero, and large surface area. The surface area is diminished somewhat because of the flexed position assumed by the SGA infant. (See "Cold Stress" in this chapter for management.)
		4. **Hypoglycemia.** High metabolic rate (secondary to heat loss), poor liver glycogen stores, and inhibited gluconeogenesis lead to low blood sugar levels.

Classification	Physical Characteristics	Clinical Problems
Small for gestational age (SGA) *(continued)*		(See "Hypoglycemia" in this chapter for management.)
		5. **Hypocalcemia.** Calcium depletion secondary to birth asphyxia.
		6. **Polycythemia.** A physiologic response to in utero chronic hypoxic stress. (See this chapter for management.)
Large for gestational age (LCA), especially infant of diabetic mother (IDM)	Appears fat and enlarged If IDM, cushingnoid facial (round face) and neck features Overall ruddiness Has enlarged liver, spleen, and heart Initially lethargic then irritable and jittery	1. **Hypoglycemia.** After birth the most common problem of an IDM is hypoglycemia. Even though the high maternal blood supply is lost, this newborn continues to produce high levels of insulin, which deplete the blood glucose within hours after birth. IDMs also have less ability to release glucagon and catecholamines, which normally stimulate glucagon breakdown and glucose release. (See "Hypoglycemia" in this chapter for management.)
		2. **Hypocalcemia.** Associated with prematurity and hyperphosphatemia or asphyxia

Classification	Physical Characteristics	Clinical Problems
Large for gestational age (LCA) *(continued)*		3. **Hyperbilirubinemia.** This condition may be seen at 48 to 72 hours after birth. It may be caused by slightly decreased extracellular fluid volume, which increases the hematocrit level. Enclosed hemorrhages resulting from complicated vaginal birth may also cause hyperbilirubinemia. There may also be an increase in rate of bilirubin production in the presence of polycythemia. (See "Jaundice" in this chapter.)

4. **Polycythemia.** This condition may be caused by the decreased extracellular volume in IDMs. Current research centers on the fact that hemoglobin A_{lc} binds oxygen, which decreases the oxygen available to the fetal tissues. This tissue hypoxia stimulates increased erythropoietin production, which increases the hematocrit level. (See "Polycythemia" in this chapter for management.)

5. **Birth injuries,** such as fractures of the clavicle, facial

Classification	Physical Characteristics	Clinical Problems
Large for gestational age (LCA) *(continued)*		nerve paralysis, Erb's paralysis, and diaphragmatic paralysis.

6. **Cephalhematoma**

7. **Respiratory distress.** This complication occurs especially in newborns of White's classes A–C diabetic mothers. Increasing evidence suggests that IDMs may have normal levels of the phospholipids that make up surfactant, which leads others to theorize that the composition of the lipids themselves is altered in the lungs of IDMs. (See "Respiratory Distress Syndrome" in this chapter.)

Classification	Physical Characteristics	Clinical Problems
Preterm infant	Color—usually pink or ruddy but may be acrocyanotic; observe for cyanosis, jaundice, pallor, or plethora	1. **Apnea.** Cessation of breathing for more than 20 seconds. It is thought to be primarily a result of neuronal immaturity, a factor that contributes to the tendency for irregular breathing patterns in preterm infants. When cyanosis and bradycardia (heart rate less than 100 beats/ min) are also present, these periods are called apneic episodes or spells
	Skin—reddened, translucent, blood vessels readily apparent, lack of subcutaneous fat	
	Lanugo—plentiful, widely distributed	
	Head size— appears large in relation to body	

Classification	Physical Characteristics	Clinical Problems
Preterm infant *(continued)*	Skull—bones pliable, fontanelle smooth and flat	2. **Patent ductus arteriosus.** Failure of ductus arteriosus to close because of decreased pulmonary arteriole musculature and hypoxemia.
	Ears—minimal cartilage, pliable, folded over	
	Nails—soft, short	3. **Respiratory distress syndrome (RDS).** Respiratory distress results from inadequate surfactant production. (See "Respiratory Distress Syndrome" in this chapter.)
	Genitals—small; testes may not be descended	
	Resting position—flaccid, froglike	
	Cry—weak, feeble	4. **Intraventricular hemorrhage.** Up to 35 weeks' gestation the preterm's brain ventricles are lined by the germinal matrix, which is highly susceptible to hypoxic events. The germinal matrix is very vascular, and these blood vessels rupture in the presence of hypoxia.
	Reflexes—poor sucking, swallowing, and gag	
	Activity—jerky, generalized movements (seizure activity is abnormal)	
		5. **Hypocalcemia.** The preterm infant lacks adequate amounts of calcium secondary to early birth and growth needs.
		6. **Hypoglycemia.** The preterm infant's decreased brown fat and glycogen stores and increased metabolic needs predispose this infant to

Classification	Physical Characteristics	Clinical Problems
Preterm infant *(continued)*		hypoglycemia. (See "Hypoglycemia" and "Cold Stress" in this chapter for management.)

7. **Necrotizing enterocolitis.** This condition occurs when blood flow to the gastrointestinal tract is decreased secondary to shock or prolonged hypoxia.

8. **Anemia.** The preterm infant is at risk for anemia because of the rapid rate of growth required, shorter red blood cell life, excessive blood sampling, decreased iron stores, and deficiency of vitamin E.

9. **Hyperbilirubinemia.** Immature hepatic enzymatic function decreases conjugation of bilirubin, resulting in increased bilirubin levels. (See "Jaundice" in this chapter.)

10. **Infection.** The preterm infant is more susceptible to infection than term infants. Most of the neonate's immunity is acquired in the last trimester.

Classification	Physical Characteristics	Clinical Problems
Preterm infant *(continued)*		Therefore the preterm infant has decreased antibodies available for protection.
Post-term infant	Generally has normal skull, but reduced dimensions of rest of body make skull look inordinately large	1. **Hypoglycemia** Nutritional deprivation and resultant depleted glycogen stores. (See "Hypoglycemia" in this chapter for management.)
	Dry, cracked skin (desquamating), parchmentlike at birth	2. **Meconium aspiration** Response to hypoxia in utero.
	Nails of hard consistency extending beyond fingertips	3. **Polycythemia** due to increased production of red blood cells (RBCs) in response to hypoxia. (See "Polycythemia" in this chapter for management.)
	Profuse scalp hair	
	Subcutaneous fat layers depleted, leaving skin loose and giving an "old person" appearance	4. **Congenital anomalies of unknown cause.**
	Long and thin body contour	5. **Seizure** activity Because of hypoxic insult.
	Absent vernix	
	Often meconium staining (golden yellow to green) of skin, nails, and cord	6. **Cold stress** because of loss or poor development of subcutaneous fat. (See "cold stress" management in this chapter.)
	May have an alert, wide-eyed appearance symptomatic of chronic intrauterine hypoxia	

HEMATOLOGIC PROBLEMS OF THE NEWBORN

Type	Characteristics	Critical Nursing Management
Anemia Term (Hb < 14 gm/dL) Preterm (Hb < 13 gm/dL)	Pale, > 5% to 10% expected weight loss in first few days of life, slow weight gain in first months of life. Tachycardia may be present. Profound tachycardia (HR > 160) seen in hemorrhage.	**Preventive:** Term baby: Provide iron-fortified formula (2 mg/kg/day). Preterm baby: Give 25 IU of vitamin E p.o. daily with feedings until baby is two to three months of age.

After two months of age switch to iron supplementation in formula.

Symptomatic newborn: (Needs increased oxygen as do growing premature infants.) Administer packed RBCs transfusion:

- Warm blood.

- Give ordered amount over > 30 min.

- Monitor for hypocalcemia and hypoglycemia.

- Don't exceed 10 mL/kg (of weight) volume per transfusion.

- Recheck Hct/Hb per agency protocol.

Type	Characteristics	Critical Nursing Management
Polycythemia Venous Hct > 65% and increased viscosity leads to impaired blood flow through blood vessels and decreased oxygen transport. LGA, IDM, SGA, and infants of pregnancy induced hypertension (PIH) mothers are at risk.	Plethoric but cyanotic when crying. Tachypnea, tachycardia, possible murmur, congenital heart failure (CHF), respiratory distress. Feeding intolerance and necrotizing enterocolitis (NEC). Hypoglycemia, lethargy, tremors, hypotonia, poor reflexes, and possible seizures secondary to decreased cerebral perfusion. Jaundice secondary to increased RBC breakdown. Microthrombi may occur in renal and cerebral artery.	Monitor pulse, respirations. Keep urine specific gravity < 1.015. Assess color at rest and when crying. Obtain capillary blood sample for Hct (warm heel prior to heel stick; this increases blood flow and mirrors central Hct). If heel stick Hct is > 65%, obtain central Hct to verify polycythemia. **If Hct > 65% but baby is asymptomatic:** Increase fluid intake by 20–40 mL/ kg/day. Recheck heel stick Hct q6hrs. **If Hct > 65% and baby is symptomatic:** Assist with partial exchange transfusion (remove some RBCs and replace with fresh frozen plasma [FFP] or 5% albumin, or normal saline). The goal is to lower Hct to 60% or less. Monitor newborn's response to the procedure: Take VS. **Be alert for:** increased P, R, and T, signs of hypoglycemia and NEC. Obtain serial Hcts after exchange as ordered.

JAUNDICE

Overview

Hyperbilirubinemia is an above normal amount of bilirubin in the blood, which, when the level is high enough, produces jaundice. Jaundice can be seen as a visible yellowing of the skin, mucosa, sclera, and urine. Physiologic jaundice is the rise and fall in the serum bilirubin (indirect) level (4 to 12 mg/dL) by the fourth day after birth and peaking by the third to fifth day. Physiologic jaundice is common in term infants and is a result of neonatal hepatic immaturity. Pathologic jaundice is marked by yellow skin discoloration and an increase in the serum bilirubin level above 12 mg/dL within 24 hours after birth. The bilirubin level rises faster than 5 mg/dL in 24 hrs and may continue beyond a week in full-term newborns and two weeks in premature infants. Pathologic jaundice is most commonly associated with blood type or blood group incompatibility, infection, or biliary, hepatic, or metabolic abnormalities.

Medical Management

Phototherapy and exchange transfusions are the primary medical treatments for hyperbilirubinemia (see Procedure 5: Exchange Transfusion: Nursing Responsibilities). Drug therapy (albumin, phenobarbital) may also be used.

Critical Nursing Assessments

1. Assess for risk factors.
   Be alert for: Prenatal history of Rh immunization, ABO incompatability, maternal use of aspirin, sulfonamides, or antimicrobial drugs; Native American, Japanese, Chinese, or Korean nationality (predisposed to higher bilirubin levels); yellow amniotic fluid, which indicates significant hemolytic disease.

2. Assess color of skin, sclera, mucous membranes.
   Assessment technique: Observe in the daylight, or, using white fluorescent lights, blanch skin over bony prominence to remove capillary coloration and then assess degree of yellow discoloration. Assess oral mucosa and conjunctival sac in dark-skinned infants.

Be alert for: In first 24 hours after birth, jaundice mandates immediate investigation. Pallor is associated with hemolytic anemia.

3. Assess laboratory results.
Be alert for: Serum bilirubin increase of 5 mg/dL/day or more than 0.5 mg/hr, or increase in cord bilirubin to 4 mg/dL indicates severe hemolysis or pathologic process. Increased reticulocytes and decreased Hct and Hbg levels are also significant.

4. Assess clinical signs and symptoms.
Be alert for: Poor feeding, lethargy, tremors, high-pitched cry, absent Moro reflex are often first signs of bilirubin encephalopathy (kernicterus). Vomiting, irritability, rigid musculature, opisthotonos, seizures are later signs of encephalopathy and may indicate permanent damage.

Sample Nursing Diagnoses

- Fluid volume deficit related to decreased intake, loose stools, and increased insensible water loss.
- Altered parenting related to interruption in bonding between infant and parents secondary to separation.
- Risk for injury related to use of phototherapy.

Critical Nursing Interventions

1. Initiate feedings as soon as possible and continue q 2–4 hrs.

While under phototherapy:

1. Place infant under phototherapy lights unclothed, except perhaps for covering of genitals, to maximize exposure to lights. Phototherapy reduces bilirubin in the skin.
Be alert for: If surgical mask is used, remove metal nose strip to prevent burns.

2. Cover infant's eyes when under the lights. Remove eye covers at least every four hours for ten minutes with phototherapy lights off. Change eye patches every 24 hours. Mark patches with time, date, and right and left eye designation (to avoid cross conta-

mination). Inspect eyes and check under the eye dressings for pressure areas.
Be alert for: High density light may cause retinal injury and corneal burns. Irritation from patches may cause corneal abrasions and conjunctivitis.

3. Monitor vital signs every four hours. If hypo/hyperthermia occurs, check temperature every hour.

4. Monitor intake and output every eight hours. Weigh infant daily (provides more accurate determination of fluid intake and insensible water loss caused by phototherapy). Determine urine specific gravities q8hrs. Notify physician if specific gravity > 1.015, an indication of dehydration.
Be alert for: Urine specific gravity results can be influenced by sugar, protein, blood, and urobiligen in the urine. Urine may be green because of the photodegradation of bilirubin. Stools are usually loose and green in color.

5. Provide fluid intake 25% above normal requirements to meet increase in insensible water losses and losses in the stools. Offer D5W p.o. between breast-feeding or formula intake.

6. Reposition infant at least every 2–4 hours. Monitor skin for excoriations, rash, or bronzing of the skin. Change diaper and clean area as soon after stooling to prevent skin breakdown.
Tip: Ongoing assessment of skin must be done with the phototherapy lights off.

7. Turn phototherapy lights off when parents visit and for feedings. Coordinate care activities with parent visits so that parents have maximum contact with their baby with the phototherapy lights off.

8. Monitor phototherapy lights' wave-length using bilimeter every shift.

9. Monitor bilirubin levels every eight hours for first one to two days or per agency protocol after discontinuation of phototherapy. Turn lights off when doing bilirubin laboratory tests. Bilirubin levels may rebound following phototherapy. **If an exchange transfusion is done:** See Procedure 5: Exchange Transfusion: Nursing Responsibilities.

Evaluation

Anticipated outcomes of nursing care include the following:

- The risks for development of hyperbilirubinemia are identified, and action is taken to minimize the potential impact of hyperbilirubinemia.
- The baby will not have any corneal irritation or drainage, skin breakdown, or major fluctuations in temperature.
- Parents will understand the rationale for, goal of, and expected outcome of therapy. Parents verbalize their concerns about their baby's condition and identify how they can facilitate their baby's improvement.

NURSING CARE NEEDS OF NEWBORNS OF SUBSTANCE-ABUSE MOTHERS

Type	Physical Characteristics	Early Neonatal Nursing Interventions
Fetal alcohol syndrome (FAS)	SGA	Monitor vital signs. Be alert for: apnea, cyanosis, and hypothermia.
	Abnormal features:	
	Microcephaly	Provide heat conservation measures, eg, cap for head, double wrap; for additional management see "Cold Stress" in this chapter.
	Craniofacial abnormalities	
	Epicanthal folds	
	Prenatal and postnatal growth defects	
	Congenital heart defects	Note feeding problems/patterns (offer small, frequent feedings).
	Mental retardation	Measure abdominal girth. Be alert for abdominal distention.
	Abnormal palmar creases	
	Withdrawal symptoms: hyperactivity, tremors, lethargy, poor suck reflex	Provide oxygen via nasal cannula or mask and bulb suction as ordered for

Type	Physical Characteristics	Early Neonatal Nursing Interventions
Fetal alcohol syndrome (FAS) *(continued)*	Can start after birth and usually subside within first 72 hours after onset	respiratory distress or aspiration.
		Place baby in dimly lit environment to prevent overstimulation.
	Potential for seizure	
Newborn of drug-dependent mother	SGA or premature	Assess ability to feed (hyperactivity and increased secretions cause difficulty). Be alert for difficult feeder with poor suck and regurgitation/vomiting. Provide small, frequent feedings.
	Withdrawal symptoms (onset varies from birth to two weeks of age): Nasal stuffiness, sneezing, yawning, increased sucking efforts, hiccups	
	Increased secretions, difficulty feeding, drooling, gagging, vomiting, diarrhea	Bulb suction newborn. Position on side with head elevated to prevent choking.
	Increased respiratory rate, shrill cry, respiratory distress	Note frequency of diarrhea and vomiting and weigh every 8 hours during withdrawal.
	Irritability, tremors, hyperactivity, hypertonia, hyperreflexia, increased Moro reflex, disturbed sleeping pattern	Initiate safety precautions to prevent baby self-injury during periods of hyperactivity. Observe for seizures.
	Seizures (infrequent, but may occur in severe cases or with intrauterine asphyxia)	Decrease stimulating activities and provide quiet environment during withdrawal period. Provide gentle handling, pacifier, talk in soothing voice, play

Type	Physical Characteristics	Early Neonatal Nursing Interventions
Newborn of drug-dependent mother *(continued)*	Fever, flushing, diaphoresis Dehydration	quiet music, swaddle snugly with hands near mouth, and hold as much as baby tolerates. Encourage parent-infant attachment by explaining baby's behavior and giving comfort suggestions. Administer drugs— phenobarbital, chlorpromazine (Thorazine), para-goric, or laudanum— as ordered for relief of withdrawal symptoms. Methadone should not be given because of possible newborn addiction to it.

CONGENITAL HEART DISEASE IN THE NEWBORN PERIOD

Overview

Congenital heart disease (CHD) occurs in about 4–5 per 1000 live births. The CHDs seen most often in the first week of life are transposition of the great vessels and hypoplastic left heart syndrome. Within the first month of life, the presenting conditions are coarctation of the aorta, ventricular septal defect, tetralogy of Fallot, and patent ductus arteriosus. Initial assessment of the newborn suspected of having CHD includes: complete physical exam, blood pressure in all four extremities, electrocardiogram (ECG), chest x-ray, and evaluation of oxygenation in 100% oxygen. Now many newborns with congenital heart disease are diagnosed by fetal echocardiography, and corrective management can be done during the first month of life.

Medical Management

Cardiac defects of the early newborn period include:

Congenital Heart Defect	Clinical Findings	Medical/Surgical Management
Patent ductus arteriosus (PDA): ↑ in females, maternal rubella, RDS, < 1500 gm preterm newborns, high-altitude births	Harsh grade 2–3 machinery murmur at upper left sternal border (LSB) just beneath clavicle ↑ difference between systolic and diastolic pulse pressure Can lead to right heart failure and pulmonary congestion ↑ left atrial (LA) and left ventricular (LV) enlargement, dilated ascending aorta ↑ pulmonary vascularity	Indomethacin— 0.2 mg/kg orally (prostaglandin inhibitor) up to 3 doses Surgical ligation/ resection Use of O_2 therapy and blood transfusion to improve tissue oxygenation and perfusion Fluid restriction and diuretics

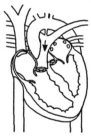

Patent ductus arteriosus.

Coarctation of aorta Can be preductal or postductal	Absent or diminished femoral pulses Increased brachial pulses Late systolic murmur in left intrascapular area Systolic BP in lower extremities	Surgical resection of narrowed portion of aorta Prostaglandin E_1 to maintain ductus open

Congenital Heart Defect	Clinical Findings	Medical/Surgical Management
Coarctation of aorta *(continued)*	Enlarged left ventricle Can present in CHF at 7–21 days of life	

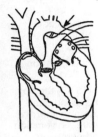

Coarctation of the aorta.

Transposition of great vessels (TGA) (↑ females, IDMs, LGAs)	Cyanosis at birth or within three days Possible pulmonic stenosis murmur Right ventricular hypertrophy Polycythemia "Egg on its side" x-ray	Prostaglandin E_1 to vasodilate ductus to keep it open Initial surgery to create opening between right and left side of heart if none exists Total surgical repair—usually the arterial switch

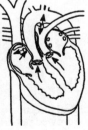

Complete transposition of great vessels. (All illustrations from Congenital Heart Abnormalities. *Clinical Education Aid no. 7. Ross Laboratories, Columbus, Ohio.)*

Hypoplastic left heart syndrome	Normal at birth— cyanosis and shock-like congestive heart failure develop within a few hours to days	Currently no effective corrective treatment (total repair) Palliative use of prostaglandin E_1.

Congenital Heart Defect	Clinical Findings	Medical/Surgical Management
Hypoplastic left heart syndrome *(continued)*	Soft systolic murmur just left of the sternum	
	Diminished pulses	
	Aortic and/or mitral atresia	
	Tiny, thick-walled left ventricle	
	Large, dilated, hypertrophied right ventricle	
	X-ray: Cardiac enlargement and pulmonary venous congestion	

Critical Nursing Assessments

Nursing assessment of the following signs and symptoms assists in identifying the newborn with a cardiac problem:

1. Tachypnea: reflects increased pulmonary blood flow

2. Dyspnea: caused by increased pulmonary venous pressure and blood flow; can also cause chest retractions, wheezing

3. Color: ashen, gray, or cyanotic

4. Difficulty in feeding: requires many rest periods before finishing even 1 or 2 ounces

5. Diaphoresis: beads of perspiration over the upper lip and forehead; may accompany feeding fatigue

6. Stridor or choking spells

7. Failure to gain weight

8. Heart murmur: may not be heard in left-to-right shunting defects because the pulmonary pressure in the newborn is greater than pressure in the left side of the heart in the early newborn period

9. Hepatomegaly: in right-sided heart failure, caused by venous congestion in the liver

10. Tachycardia: pulse over 160, may be as high as 200

11. Cardiac enlargement

Sample Nursing Diagnoses

- Altered tissue perfusion related to decrease in circulating oxygen.
- Ineffective breathing pattern related to fatigue.
- Altered nutrition: less than body requirements related to increased energy expenditure.
- Knowledge deficit related to lack of information about cardiac anomaly and future implications for care.

Critical Nursing Interventions

1. Give small, frequent feedings (oral), or gastric tube feeding to conserve energy (see Procedure 9: Gavage Feeding).

2. Obtain daily weights and strict intake and output. **Be alert for:** Failure to gain weight, inability to take more than an ounce of formula in 30–45 min of feeding, and decrease in urine output. Also note weight gain reflected as body edema.

3. Provide oxygen to relieve respiratory distress and keep oxygen level at 30% to 40%. Oxygen will not remove cyanosis.

4. Administer digoxin per order. Dosage should be double-checked by a second RN. It is given only after listening to the apical pulse for one minute and if no irregularities or slowing are noted. **Tip:** In most agencies, if pulse is lower than 120 bpm, check with physician before giving medication.

5. Diuretics (such as furosemide) are administered; potassium levels should be monitored because diuretics cause excretion of potassium.

6. Morphine sulfate, 0.05 mg/kg of body weight per dose, may be given for irritability. It decreases peripheral and pulmonary resistance, and therefore decreases tachypnea. Place in semi-Fowler's position to ease breathing.

7. Fentanyl provides good pain control without respiratory depression seen with morphine sulfate.

8. Counsel parents on home care: administration of drugs, indications of drug toxicity, and measures used to prevent fatigue and promote nutrition for growth and development.

Evaluation

- Newborn's oxygen consumption and energy expenditure are minimal while at rest and during feedings.
- Newborn is protected from additional stresses such as infection, cold stress, and dehydration.
- Parents verbalize their concerns about their baby's health maintenance and need for ongoing follow-up care.

CONGENITAL ANOMALIES: IDENTIFICATION AND CARE IN NEWBORN PERIOD

Congenital Anomaly	Nursing Assessments	Nursing Goals and Interventions
Congenital hydrocephalus (1 in 1200 live births)	Enlarged head	Assess presence of hydrocephalus: Measure and plot occipital-frontal baseline measurements, then measure head circumference once a day.
	Enlarged or full fontanelles	
	Split or widened sutures	
	"Setting sun" eyes	
	Head circumference >90% on growth chart	Check fontanelle for bulging and sutures for widening.
		Assist with head ultrasound and transillumination
		Maintain skin integrity: Change position frequently.
		Clean skin creases after feeding or vomiting.

Congenital Anomaly	Nursing Assessments	Nursing Goals and Interventions
Congenital hydrocephalus *(continued)*		Use sheepskin pillow under head.
		Postoperatively, position head off operative site.
		Watch for signs of infection.
Choanal atresia	Occlusion of posterior nares	Assess patency of nares: Listen for breath sounds while holding baby's mouth closed and alternately compressing each nostril.
	Cyanosis and retractions at rest	
	Snorting respirations	
	Difficulty breathing during feeding	Assist with passing feeding tube to confirm diagnosis.
	Obstruction by thick mucus	Maintain respiratory function: Assist with taping airway in mouth to prevent respiratory distress.
		Position with head elevated to improve air exchange.
Cleft lip (1 in 850–1000 live births)	Unilateral or bilateral visible defect	Provide nutrition: Feed with special nipple.
	May involve external nares, nasal cartilage, nasal septum, and alveolar process	Burp frequently (increased tendency to swallow air and reflex vomiting).
	Flattening or depression of midfacial contour	Clean cleft with sterile water (to prevent crusting on cleft prior to repair).

Congenital Anomaly	Nursing Assessments	Nursing Goals and Interventions
Cleft lip *(continued)*		Support parental coping: Assist parents with grief over loss of idealized baby.
		Encourage verbalization of their feelings about visible defect.
		Provide role model in interacting with infant. (Parents internalize others' responses to their newborn.)
Cleft palate (1 in 2500 live births)	Fissure connecting oral and nasal cavity	Prevent aspiration/infection: Place prone or in side-lying position to facilitate drainage.
	May involve uvula and soft palate	Suction nasopharyngeal cavity (to prevent aspiration or airway obstruction).
	May extend forward to nostril, involving hard palate and maxillary alveolar ridge	During neonatal period, feed in upright position with head and chest tilted slightly backward (to aid swallowing and discourage aspiration)
	Difficulty in sucking	Provide nutrition. Feed with special nipple that fills cleft and allows sucking. Also decreases chance of aspiration through nasal cavity.
	Expulsion of formula through nose	

Congenital Anomaly	Nursing Assessments	Nursing Goals and Interventions
Cleft palate *(continued)*		Clean mouth with water after feedings.
		Burp after each ounce (tend to swallow large amounts of air).
		Thicken formula to provide extra calories.
		Plot weight gain patterns to assess adequacy of diet.
		Provide parental support: Refer parents to community agencies and support groups. Encourage verbalization of frustrations as feeding process is long and frustrating.
		Praise all parental efforts.
		Encourage parents to seek prompt treatment for upper respiratory infection (URI) and teach them ways to decrease URI.
Tracheoesophageal fistula (type 3) (1 in 3500 live births)	History of maternal hydramnios	Maintain respiratory status and prevent aspiration. Withhold feeding until esophageal patency is determined.
	Excessive mucous secretions	
	Constant drooling	Quickly assess patency before putting to breast in birth area.
	Abdominal distention beginning soon after birth	

Congenital Anomaly	Nursing Assessments	Nursing Goals and Interventions
Tracheoesophageal fistula (Type 3) *(continued)*	Periodic choking and cyanotic episodes	Place on low intermittent suction to control saliva and mucus (to prevent aspiration pneumonia).
	Immediate regurgitation of feeding	Place in warmed, humidified Isolette (liquefies secretions, facilitating removal).
	Clinical symptoms of aspiration pneumonia (tachypnea, retractions, rhonchi, decreased breath sounds, cyanotic spells)	Elevate head of bed 20°–40° (to prevent reflux of gastric juices).
	Failure to pass nasogastric tube	Keep quiet (crying causes air to pass through fistula and to distend intestines, causing respiratory embarrassment).
		Maintain fluid and electrolyte balance: Give fluids to replace esophageal drainage and maintain hydration.
		Provide parent education: Explain staged repair: provision of gastrostomy and ligation of fistula, then repair of atresia.
		Keep parents informed; clarify and reinforce physician's explanations regarding malformation, surgical repair, pre- and postoperative care, and prognosis.

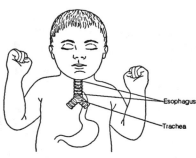

Esophagus

Trachea

Figure 6–2 *The most frequently seen type of congenital tracheoesophageal fistula and esophageal atresia.*

Congenital Anomaly	Nursing Assessments	Nursing Goals and Interventions
Tracheoeso- phageal fistula (Type 3) *(continued)*		Involve parents in care of infant and in planning for future; facilitate touch and eye contact (to dispel feelings of inadequacy, increase self-esteem and self-worth, and promote incorporation of infant into family).
Diaphragmatic hernia (1 in 4000 live births	Difficulty initiating respirations	Maintain respiratory status: Immediately administer oxygen.
	Gasping respirations with nasal flaring and chest retraction	Never ventilate with a mask and bag and O_2 because stomach will inflate further, compressing the lungs.
	Barrel chest and scaphoid abdomen	Initiate gastric decompression.
	Asymmetric chest expansion	Place in high semi-Fowler's position (to use gravity to keep abdominal organ's pressure off diaphragm).
	Breath sounds may be absent, usually on left side	
	Heart sounds displaced to right	Turn to affected side to allow unaffected lung expansion.
	Spasmodic attacks of cyanosis and difficulty in feeding	Carry out interventions to alleviate respiratory and metabolic acidosis.
	Bowel sounds may be heard in thoracic cavity	Assess for increased secretions around suction tube (denotes possible obstruction).

Congenital Anomaly	Nursing Assessments	Nursing Goals and Interventions
Diaphragmatic hernia *(continued)*		Aspirate and irrigate tube with air or sterile water.
Omphalocele (1 in 6000–10,000 live births)	Herniation of abdominal contents into base of umbilical cord	Maintain hydration and temperature: Provide D_5LR and albumin for hypovolemia.
	May have an enclosed transparent sac covering	Place infant in sterile bag up to above defect.
		Cover sac with moistened sterile gauze and place plastic wrap over dressing (to prevent rupture of sac and infection).
		Initiate gastric decompression by insertion of nasogastric tube attached to low suction (to prevent distention of lower bowel and impairment of blood flow).
		Prevent infection and trauma to defect.
		Position to prevent trauma to defect.
		Administer broad-spectrum antibiotics.
Myelomeningocele (0.5 in 1000 live births)	Saclike cyst containing meninges, spinal cord, and nerve roots in thoracic and/or lumbar area	Prevent trauma and infection.
		Position on abdomen or on side and restrain

Congenital Anomaly	Nursing Assessments	Nursing Goals and Interventions
Myelomeningo-cele *(continued)*	Myelomeningocele directly connects to subarachnoid space so hydrocephalus often associated	(to prevent pressure and trauma to sac).
	No response or varying response to sensation below level of sac	Meticulously clean buttocks and genitals after each voiding and defecation (to prevent contamination of sac and decrease possibility of infection).
	May have constant dribbling of urine	May put protective covering over sac (to prevent rupture and drying).
	Incontinence or retention of stool	Observe sac for oozing of fluid or pus.
	Anal opening may be flaccid	Use the Credé method to express urine from bladder (apply downward pressure on bladder with thumbs moving urine toward the urethra) as ordered to prevent urinary stasis.
		Assess amount of sensation and movement below defect.
		Observe for complications: Obtain occipital-frontal circumference baseline measurements, then measure head circumference once a day (to detect hydrocephalus).
		Check fontanelle for bulging.

Congenital Anomaly	Nursing Assessments	Nursing Goals and Interventions
Congenital dislocated hip (1 in 200 live births)	Asymmetric gluteal and anterior thigh fold	Maintain abduction position via Pavik harness or plastic abduction splint.
	One leg may be shorter	Provide good perineal care to prevent skin breakdown.
	Positive Ortolani test (clunk noted with gentle forced abduction of leg and palpable bulge of head of femur)	Instruct parents on home care of appliance.
Clubfoot (1 in 1000 live births)	Abnormal turning of foot/feet either inward or outward	If casted, keep casts dry, protect legs from irritation. Carry out circulatory and neurologic checks.
	Unable to rotate to normal position	Soothe infant during and after castings.
		Provide parents with cast-care instructions (handling, cleaning, and signs of complications).
Imperforate anus (1 in 5000 live births)	Visible anal membrane	Monitor passage of first stool.
	Absence of patent anus	Take axillary temperature.
	Inability to take rectal temperature	Measure abdominal girth (increasing abdominal distention).
	No passage of meconium	Prepare parents for possible need for temporary colostomy.
	Abdominal distention	

PERINATALLY ACQUIRED NEWBORN INFECTIONS

Infection	Critical Nursing Assessments	Critical Nursing Interventions
Group B streptococcus 1% to 2% colonized with one in ten developing disease Early onset— usually within hours of birth or within first week Late onset— one week to three months	Assess for risk factors, eg, low Apgar scores Assess for: Severe respiratory distress (grunting and cyanosis) May become apneic or demonstrate symptoms of shock Meconium-stained amniotic fluid seen at birth	Closely monitor VS for signs of respiratory distress and infection. Assist with x-ray— shows aspiration pneumonia or respiratory distress syndrome. Immediately obtain blood, gastric aspirate, external ear canal, and nasopharynx cultures. Administer antibiotics, usually aqueous penicillin or ampicillin combined with gentamicin as soon as cultures are obtained. Initiate referral to evaluate for blindness, deafness, learning or behavioral problems.
***Escherichia coli* K1 (ECK1)** 2nd most common cause of newborn sepsis/meningitis. Incidence 1% to 2% of live births	Assess for: seven to ten green, watery stools/day Dehydration, electrolyte imbalances, sepsis	Institute infection-control measures. Isolate from other babies. Strict hand washing. Weigh at least daily. Maintain hydration by IV/PO. Administer antibiotics per order.

Infection	Critical Nursing Assessments	Critical Nursing Interventions
Gonorrhea Approximately 30%–35% of newborns born vaginally to infected mothers are infected. Onset 7–14 days after birth	Assess for: Ophthalmia neonatorum (conjunctivitis) Purulent discharge and corneal ulcerations Neonatal sepsis with temperature instability, poor feeding response, and/or hypotonia, jaundice	Administer 1% silver nitrate solution or ophthalmic antibiotic ointment (see Drug Guide: Erythromycin [Ilotycin] ophthalmic ointment), or 1% tetracycline ointment. May give aqueous penicillin G IM as ordered if mother's culture positive. Maintain body substance isolation during procedures, educate parents regarding need for careful hand washing, etc. Initiate follow-up referral to evaluate any loss of vision.
Chlamydia trachomatis Acquired during passage through birth canal Appears 5–14 days after birth	Assess for perinatal history of preterm birth Symptomatic newborns present with pneumonia—conjunctivitis (purulent yellow discharge and eyelid swelling) after three to four days Chronic follicular conjunctivitis (corneal neovascularization and conjunctival scarring)	Maintain body substance isolation. Obtain smears for cultures as ordered. Administer erythromycin p.o. and topical 10% sulfonamide drops. Wash eyes with warmed normal saline solution as needed. Initiate follow-up referral for eye complications and late development of pneumonia at 4–11 weeks postnatally.

Infection	Critical Nursing Assessments	Critical Nursing Interventions
Herpes type 2 1 in 75,000 live births. Usually transmitted during vaginal birth	Assess for: Small cluster vesicular skin lesions over all the body Check perinatal history for active herpes genital lesions Disseminated form—DIC, pneumonia, hepatitis with jaundice, hepatosplenomegaly; and neurologic abnormalities. Without skin lesions, see fever or subnormal temperature, respiratory congestion, tachypnea, and tachycardia.	Carry out careful hand washing and gown and glove isolation with linen precautions. Administer intravenous vidarabine (Vira A) or acyclovir (Zovirax). Initiate follow-up referral to evaluate potential sequelae of microcephaly, spasticity, seizures, deafness, or blindness. Encourage parental rooming-in and touching of their newborn. Show parents appropriate hand washing procedures and precautions to be used at home if mother's lesions are active. Obtain throat, conjunctiva, cerebral spinal fluid (CSF), blood, urine, and lesion cultures to identify herpesvirus type 2 antibodies in serum IgM fraction. Cultures positive in 24-48 hours.
AIDS (placental transmission)	Assess mother for risk factors: HIV-positive, infected sexual partners, drug use, or needle sharing.	Take vital signs q4hrs. Provide meticulous skin care and change diaper after each voiding and stooling.

Infection	Critical Nursing Assessments	Critical Nursing Interventions
AIDS *(continued)*	Assess for S & S of opportunistic infections, failure to thrive, weight loss, > 3 diarrheal stools/day, feeding intolerance, diaper rash, hepatosplenomegaly, anemia, respiratory difficulty, lethargy, temperature instability, generalized skin rash, and lymphadenopathy	Maintain universal precautions per agency. See Essential Precautions in Practice in this chapter.
		Provide small, frequent feedings.
		Monitor stools for amount, type, consistency, change in patterns, occult blood, and reducing substances.
		Avoid giving infant any injections, drawing blood, or instilling eye medication until initial bath with soap and water.
	Assess skin for breakdown or rashes	Instruct woman/family on newborn health needs and need for frequent position changes.
	Assess cause of parental fear	Determine parental understanding of AIDS
		Provide emotional support to mother/family if breastfeeding was desired.
		Provide list of contact persons for available community resources and information about current and experimental treatment

Infection	Critical Nursing Assessments	Critical Nursing Interventions
Oral candida infection (thrush) Acquired during passage through birth canal	Assess buccal mucosa, tongue, gums, and inside the cheeks for white plaques (seen five to seven days of age).	Differentiate white plaque areas from milk curds by using cotton tip applicator (if it is thrush, removal of white areas causes raw bleeding areas).
	Check diaper area for bright red, well-demarcated eruptions.	Maintain cleanliness of hands, linen, clothing, diapers, and feeding apparatus.
	Assess for thrush periodically when newborn is on long-term antibiotic therapy.	Instruct breastfeeding mothers on treating their nipples with nystatin.
		Administer gentian violet (1% to 2%) swabbed on oral lesions one hour after feeding, or nystatin instilled in baby's oral cavity and on mucosa.
		Swab skin lesions with topical nystatin.
		Discuss with parents that gentian violet stains mouth and clothing.
		Avoid placing gentian violet on normal mucosa; causes irritation.

CHAPTER 7

The Postpartum Client

OVERVIEW

The period of time (approximately six weeks) following childbirth, during which the body returns to a prepregnant state, is called the puerperium. Because of current practice some women may be discharged as early as 4 hours following birth, while in most cases women are discharged within one day. Nursing care during this time focuses on assessment for developing complications and on client teaching. The nurse should use every opportunity to explain the normal physiologic changes to the woman so that she will be able to recognize deviations and contact her care giver if complications arise.

Table 7–1 identifies the basic assessments that the postpartum nurse should make, explains postpartum physiologic changes, and identifies basic teaching that is indicated.

NURSING INTERVENTIONS FOR POSTPARTUM DISCOMFORT

Perineal Discomfort: Episiotomy and Hemorrhoids

Suggested nursing interventions for the first few hours after birth include:

1. Ice glove or chemical ice bag on the perineal area. If glove is used, wash it first to remove powder, then wrap it in a washcloth or towel. Leave on 20 minutes, then off ten minutes.

Text continues on page 205

Table 7–1 Postpartum Assessment and Teaching

Physiologic Changes	Nursing Assessment	Client Teaching
Vital Signs		
Temperature: normal range; may increase to 100.4F (38C) because of exertion and mild dehydration.	Normal: 98–100.4F (36.2–38C) After first 24 hours temperature > 100.4F (38C) suggests infection.	Advise woman that following discharge, if she experiences chills, malaise, etc, she should take her temperature and report fever to her care giver.
Pulse: Puerperal bradycardia may occur for six to ten days postpartum because of decreased blood volume and cardiac strain, and increased stroke volume.	Pulse: 50–90 beats/min. Tachycardia may result from difficult labor and birth or from hemorrhage. Assess for additional signs of hemorrhage.	Explain that pulse slows normally. Advise woman to report palpitations, rapid pulse.
Respirations: unchanged	Respirations normally 16–24/min. If decreased, evaluate for medication effects; if marked tachypnea present, assess for signs of pneumonia or other respiratory disease.	Advise woman to report symptoms of complications, including difficulty breathing, cough, rapid respirations.
Blood pressure (BP): remains consistent with baseline BP. A slight	BP elevated: Consider pregnancy-induced hypertension (PIH), especially	Explain findings to woman.

decrease may indicate normal physiologic readjustment to decreased intrapelvic pressure.

if accompanied by headache (see Chapter 2). Note proteinuria, edema. BP decreased: Evaluate for additional signs of hemorrhage (rapid pulse, clammy skin).

Breasts

Immediately after birth, breasts are smooth, soft, and show changes in pigmentation, presence of striae, etc, characteristic of pregnancy.

Anterior pituitary secretion of prolactin promotes milk production by stimulating alveolar cells of breast. Oxytocin, produced by posterior pituitary when infant suckles, promotes milk letdown reflex and flow of milk results. At this time breasts are producing colostrum, which is creamy and high in maternal antibodies. By two to four days after birth, the breast begins producing milk. Breasts tend to become full and hard due to milk production and venous congestion. This is called engorgement.

Assess fit and support provided by bra, which should hold all the breast tissue, and, for breastfeeding women, have cotton straps that don't stretch. Nursing bras have flaps that open for breastfeeding.

Assess size and shape of breasts (one breast often larger than the other).

Palpate and note whether breast is soft (initially), somewhat firm (associated with filling), firm (full of milk), or hard (engorgement). Note tenderness, palpable mass, heat, edema (suggest caked breast or mastitis). If present, assess for other signs of infection, including fever, malaise.

Assess nipples for fissures, cracks, soreness, inversion.

Discuss importance of wearing a well-fitting bra 24 hours a day until breast milk is suppressed in non-nursing mother, or until breastfeeding mother stops nursing.

Discuss methods for relieving discomfort of engorgement for non-nursing and nursing mothers as indicated. (See "Breast Engorgement in the Non-nursing Mother" in this chapter, and Table 7–2.)

Review signs of infection.

Continued

Table 7–1 continued

Physiologic Changes	Nursing Assessment	Client Teaching
Abdomen		
Abdominal wall is stretched; appears loose and flabby for some time. Tone can improve in two to three months with exercise. Diastasis recti abdominis is a separation of the rectus abdominis muscle so that a portion of abdominal wall has no muscular support.	Abdomen feels soft, may have a "doughy" texture. Palpate rectus abdominis muscle, which should be intact. If a separation is felt, determine its length and width. If difficult to determine, ask woman to elevate her head, which causes tightening of the abdominal muscle.	Discuss exercises that can be done to improve tone. (See discussion on p. 216 and Figure 7–3.)
Uterus		
Involution: rapid reduction in size of the uterus and its return to a near prepregnant size following childbirth. Involution is enhanced by an uncomplicated birth, breastfeeding, and early ambulation. Immediately following expulsion of the placenta, uterus is contracted, about the size of a large grapefruit, located midway between	See Procedure 8: Fundal Assessment for correct technique. Fundus should be firm and in the midline. Displacement to the side may be caused by a full bladder. A fundus that is not firm is called "boggy." This may be caused by pressure from a full bladder, by the presence of clots, or because of diminished contractility in a woman who	Teach mother to evaluate her fundus herself. If it is boggy she can then massage it until it is firm and report this to the nurse. Explain the importance of voiding regularly to avoid pressure on the uterus.

symphysis and umbilicus. It gradually rises up to the level of the umbilicus as blood collects and forms clots within the uterus. It stays there for about one day, then decreases in size about one fingerbreadth/day. Within ten days to two weeks it is again a pelvic organ. Muscles stay contracted to clamp off blood vessels at placental site to prevent hemorrhage.

Uterine ligaments are still stretched so uterus is moveable and can be displaced by a full bladder.

Placental site takes up to six weeks to heal. Healing occurs by exfoliation so that no scar is formed, which would limit area available for future placental implantation.

has borne several children. Massage fundus gently with the fingertips until firm; if the uterus does not contract, more vigorous massage may be necessary; assess bladder for distention and have woman void if necessary; **attempt to express clots only when the uterus is firm; do not attempt to express clots from a boggy uterus.** This could cause uterine inversion. If bogginess remains or returns, notify physician or nurse-midwife. Note height of uterus in relation to umbilicus and chart. For example: Uterus firm, in the midline 1 FB U.

Lochia

After birth the uterus rids itself of the debris that remains by discharging lochia. **Lochia rubra,** which lasts for two to three days, is dark red, like menstrual flow. **Lochia serosa** lasts

Assess lochia for character, amount, odor (should have a slightly musty but not offensive odor, foul odor suggests infection), and the presence of clots. A few small clots are normal, but large

Instruct woman not to use tampons postpartum because of risk of infection. Perineal pads are generally used with a sanitary belt. (Adhesive-backed *Continued*

Table 7-1 continued

Physiologic Changes	Nursing Assessment	Client Teaching
from about the 3rd to 10th day. It is similar to serosanguineous drainage. **Lochia alba**, the final discharge, is a creamy brownish or yellowish discharge. When it stops the cervix is considered closed and risk of ascending infection is decreased. Lochia tends to be more abundant on arising (probably because of pooling in the vagina during the night). The amount may also increase with breastfeeding (oxytocin, released with suckling, stimulates uterine contraction) and with exertion. The type, amount, and consistency of lochia indicate the degree of healing of the placental site. Persistent lochia rubra or a return to rubra from serosa may indicate subinvolution or late postpartal hemorrhage.	clots are abnormal and should be investigated. Flow should never exceed moderate amount, eg, four to eight perineal pads daily. If woman reports heavy bleeding, have woman apply clean pad and reassess in one hour. If she reports passage of clots, ask her to save all pads with clots and not flush toilet if clots are expelled with urination. If accurate assessment of blood loss is necessary, weigh pads after first balancing scale with a clean, dry pad. One gram is considered equivalent to 1 mL blood. Chart amount, followed by character. For example: Lochia: small amount, rubra, no clots.	pads that are placed inside the panties move more when the woman walks and may spread contamination from the anal area to the episiotomy and vaginal opening.) Many young women have never worn a belt and may need assistance the first time. (Some agencies instead use a snug mesh panty that holds the pad in place.) Explain the progression of lochia from rubra to serosa to alba. Instruct the woman to save and report excessive clots and heavily saturated pads. She should also report failure of lochia to progress from rubra to serosa or a return to rubra from serosa. Teach woman to change pads with each voiding or bowel movement and after showering or use of a sitz bath.

Perineum

Following birth the soft tissue of the perineum may be edematous and bruised. Episiotomy may be present. Woman may also have some hemorrhoids as a result of pushing during labor.

Perineum should appear intact; slight edema and bruising normal. Marked fullness, bruising, and pain may indicate hematoma and require further evaluation.

Inspect episiotomy. There should be no **r**edness, **e**dema, **e**cchymosis, **d**rainage, and the edges should be well **a**pproximated (the acronym REEDA can help you recall these criteria). If present, they may indicate infection.

If hemorrhoids are present, they should be small and nontender; full, reddened, inflamed hemorrhoids are painful and require comfort measures (see "Perineal Discomfort: Episiotomy and Hemorrhoids" in this chapter).

The woman may apply an ice glove or pack initially to prevent edema. Teach woman to use a perineal bottle filled with warm water or a surgigator after each voiding to wash the perineum and promote healing. Teach importance of wiping from the front (urinary meatus) to the back (anal area) to prevent contamination of the episiotomy from the anal area. Teach comfort measures for hemorrhoids.

Urinary Tract

Urinary output greatly increases in the early postpartum period because of diuresis. Woman may have difficulty voiding because of decreased bladder

Assess voiding; woman should be voiding sufficient quantities (at least 250–300 mL) every four to six hours; ask about symptoms of urinary tract

Explain the importance of adequate voiding; help woman with difficulty by providing privacy, suggesting she pour
Continued

Table 7-1 continued

Physiologic Changes	Nursing Assessment	Client Teaching
sensation, swelling and bruising of tissues around urethra, increased bladder capacity, and difficulty voiding while recumbent.	infection (UTI) (urgency, frequency, dysuria); note whether bladder is palpable; determine whether fundus is in the midline. Palpate costovertebral angle (CVA) for tenderness.	warm water over perineum, encouraging ambulation, and describing visualization techniques. Identify symptoms of UTI; explain importance of adequate fluid intake (at least 2000 mL) daily.
Lower Extremities		
Stasis of blood in legs due to positioning, trauma to blood vessels, and use of stirrups, etc, increases risk of thrombophlebitis.	Inspect legs for redness, edema. Assess for Homans' sign (pain in calf when foot sharply dorsiflexed); palpate for tenderness, warmth.	Stress the importance of early ambulation to promote venous return. Encourage woman to avoid crossing legs or using knee-gatch position on bed.
Bowel Elimination		
Bowels tend to be sluggish because of lingering effects of progesterone, decreased abdominal muscle tone, and lack of food and fluid. Woman may fear bowel movement will he painful because of episiotomy, hemorrhoids, etc.	Ask woman about bowel elimination. She should have a normal bowel movement by second or third day after birth. Stool softeners may be indicated if hemorrhoids or episiotomy increase possibility of discomfort.	Explain importance of bowel elimination. Encourage ambulation, increased fluid intake, diet high in roughage. Explain risks of constipation.

Suggested nursing interventions after first few hours:

1. Sitz bath, usually ordered for 20 minutes TID or QID and PRN. It is soothing and cleansing, and its warmth promotes healing. **Note:** Some research suggests that a cool sitz bath may be more effective in reducing perineal edema. Offer women a choice of temperature.

   Procedure: Clean tub. Add water 102–105F. Place a towel in the bottom and, if it is a standard sitz tub, drape a towel over the edge to cushion the woman's legs. Woman can sit in sitz tub with hospital gown draped over the edge of the tub to provide privacy and prevent chilling. She should remain in the sitz bath for about 20 miuntes. Some tubs have a temperature control lever that permits the water to run with a stable temperature. In such cases leave the water running and open the drain. This creates a

---

Essential Precautions in Practice

During Postpartal Care

Examples of times when disposable gloves should be worn include the following:

- Assessing the perineum and lochia.
- Changing perineal pads and chux.
- Assessing the breast if there is leakage of colostrum or milk.
- Handling used breast pads.
- Handling used clothing, chux, perineal pads, and/or bedding contaminated with lochia.

Applying ice packs or topical anesthetic sprays to the perineum (although an ice pack or anesthetic spray could be applied in such a manner that contact with the perineum and a perineal pad is avoided, it is best to have gloves on so that you could assist with removal of the pad if needed).

REMEMBER to wash your hands prior to putting the disposable gloves on and again immediately after you remove the gloves.

For further information consult OSHA and CDC guidelines.

whirlpool effect. Warm, moist environment may make woman faint, so check on her frequently and have a call light available.

Disposable sitz tubs fit over a toilet with raised lid. At home the woman can fill a tub with 4 to 6 inches of water at a comfortable (not too hot) temperature. She should not bathe in the sitz tub because of the risk of introducing infection.

2. A perineal heat lamp provides dry heat to increase circulation, dry tissues, and promote healing. In current practice, heat lamps are used only occasionally because of the risk of burns. Usually used for 20 minutes TID PRN. Perineum should be cleansed first to prevent drying of secretions and to remove any ointments or sprays. Woman lies on the bed with her knees flexed and her legs spread apart. Use a 60-watt bulb and place lamp about 12–18 inches from perineum. The sheet can be draped over the woman's knees to provide privacy. **Never** place the lamp on the floor between uses.

3. Topical agents such as Dermoplast aerosol spray or Nupercainal ointment may be applied by the woman following a sitz bath. She should **not** use them before a heat lamp treatment because of the danger of tissue burn.

The above treatments are effective for episiotomy and hemorrhoids. In addition, suggested nursing interventions for hemorrhoids include the following:

1. Encourage side-lying position.

2. Teach the woman to reinsert hemorrhoids digitally. To do this she should lie on her side, place lubricant on her finger, and apply steady gentle pressure against the hemorrhoids, pushing them inside. She should hold them in place for 1 to 2 minutes then withdraw her finger. The anal sphincter should then hold them in place. She should maintain the side-lying position for a period of time.

3. Witch hazel pads may be placed against the hemorrhoids and held in place by the perineal pad. They are soothing and cool.

4. Encourage actions that help prevent constipation such as increased fluid intake, roughage in diet, early ambulation, use of stool softeners as prescribed.

Afterpains

Afterpains are the result of intermittent uterine contractions and are more common in multiparas, women who had a multiple pregnancy, and women who had hydramnios. They may be intensified by breastfeeding because oxytocin is released when the baby suckles. Suggested nursing interventions:

1. Have woman lie prone with small pillow under abdomen. This places constant pressure on the uterus, causing it to remain contracted. Tell her the pain will be intensified for a few minutes but then will subside.

2. Administer analgesic as needed. For breastfeeding women, administer about one hour before scheduled feeding.

Postpartum Diaphoresis

Diaphoresis results as the body works to eliminate excess fluid and waste. It frequently occurs at night, and the woman awakens drenched with perspiration. Suggested nursing interventions:

1. Protect woman from chilling by changing bedding and providing a fresh gown.

2. Encourage a shower (unless cultural practices forbid it).

3. Prevent thirst by offering fluids as the woman desires.

Discomfort from Immobility

The woman may have muscular aches from pushing or from spending time in stirrups. Suggested nursing interventions:

1. Encourage early ambulation. The woman may be light-headed initially because of blood loss, fatigue, medication, etc, so the nurse should assist her the first few times. This is especially important during the first shower or sitz bath, when heat may add to the problem. Stay close, have a call light and chair readily available, and check the woman frequently.

Suppression of Lactation in the Non-Nursing Mother

Lactation may be suppressed through mechanical inhibition.

Mechanical suppression:

1. Have the woman wear a well-fitting supportive bra continuously until lactation is suppressed (about five days). The bra is removed only for showers. A breast binder may be applied if the woman prefers or if no bra is available.

2. Apply ice packs over axillary area of both breasts for 20 minutes QID.

3. Avoid any stimulation of breasts by the woman, her partner, or infant.

4. Avoid warmth, which stimulates milk production; avoid letting shower water flow over breasts.

Breast Engorgement in the Non-Nursing Mother

1. Interventions are the same as those for suppression.

2. Administer analgesics as necessary.

Note: In the nursing mother engorgement is handled differently. See Table 7–2.

INFANT FEEDING

Breastfeeding

The hormone prolactin, from the anterior pituitary, is initially responsible for milk production, whereas oxytocin, from the posterior pituitary, is responsible for the letdown reflex, which triggers the flow of milk. The letdown reflex is stimulated by infant suckling, but it can also be stimulated by the newborn's presence or cry, or even thinking about the infant. It may also occur during sexual orgasm because oxytocin is released. The letdown reflex may be inhibited by a mother's lack of self-confidence, feelings of fear or embarrassment, or physical discomfort.

Table 7–2 Self-Care Measures for the Woman with Breastfeeding Problems

Nipple Inversion

Use Hoffman's exercises to increase protractility.

Use special breast shields such as Woolrich or Eschmann.

Use hand to shape nipple when beginning to nurse.

Apply ice for a few minutes prior to feeding to improve nipple erection.

Use electric or hand pump to cause nipple prominence, express a few drops of breast milk, then switch to regular nursing.

Inadequate Letdown

Massage breasts prior to nursing.

Feed in a quiet, private place, away from distraction.

Take a warm shower before nursing to relax and stimulate letdown.

Apply warm pack for 20 minutes before nursing.

Use relaxation techniques and focus on letdown.

Drink water, juice, or noncaffeinated beverages before and during feeding.

Avoid overfatigue by resting when the baby sleeps, feeding while lying down, and having quiet time alone.

Develop a conditioned response by establishing a routine for starting feedings.

Allow the baby sufficient time (at least 10–15 minutes per side) to trigger the letdown reflex.

Use breast-alternating method (either use different breast for each feeding or switch breasts several times during a single feeding).

If all else fails obtain a prescription for oxytocin nasal spray from the health care provider.

Nipple Soreness

Ensure that infant is correctly positioned at the breast with the infant's ear, shoulder, and hip in straight alignment.

Rotate breastfeeding positions.   *Continued*

Table 7–2   continued

Use finger to break suction before removing infant from the breast.

Hold baby close when feeding to avoid undue pulling on nipple.

Don't allow baby to sleep with nipple in mouth.

Nurse more frequently.

Begin nursing on less sore breast.

Apply ice to nipples and areola for a few minutes prior to feeding.

Protect nipples to prevent skin breakdown.

Clean nipple gently with warm water.

Allow nipples to air dry, or dry nipples with hair dryer set to low heat, or expose nipples to sunlight initially for 30 seconds, then increase to three minutes.

If clothing rubs nipples, use ventilated shields to keep clothing away from skin.

To promote healing, apply a small amount of breast milk to nipple and areola after nursing and allow to dry.

The routine application of ointment to nipple, areola, or breast (eg, lanolin, Massé cream, Eucerin cream, or A & D ointment) should be discouraged.

Apply tea bags soaked in warm water.

Change breast pads frequently.

Nurse long enough to empty breasts completely.

Alternate breasts several times during feedings.

Cracked Nipples

Use interventions discussed under sore nipples.

Inspect nipples carefully for cracks or fissures.

Temporarily stop nursing on the affected breast and hand express milk for a day or two until cracks heal.

Maintain healthy diet. Protein and vitamin C are essential for healing.

Use a mild PO analgesic such as acetaminophen for discomfort 20–30 minutes before feedings.

Continued

Table 7–2   continued

Consult health care providers if signs of infection develop.

Nipple shield should be tried before nursing on a breast is permanently discontinued, but it should be used only as a last resort. Some women find it contributes to their discomfort. Consult a lactation specialist prior to use.

Breast Engorgement

Nurse frequently (every 1–1/2 to 3 hours) around the clock.

Wear a well-fitting supportive bra at all times.

Take a warm shower or apply warm compresses to trigger letdown.

Massage breasts and then hand express some milk to soften the breast so the infant can "latch on."

Breastfeed long enough to empty breast.

Alternate starting breast.

Take a mild analgesic 20 minutes before feeding if discomfort is pronounced.

Plugged Ducts (Caked Breasts)

Nurse frequently and for long enough to empty the breasts completely.

Rotate feeding position.

Massage breasts prior to feeding, in a warm shower when possible.

Maintain good nutrition and adequate fluid intake.

Milk production is based on the law of supply and demand. Repeated inhibition of the letdown reflex or failure to empty the breasts completely and frequently may decrease milk supply.

Breastfeeding technique

1. Put the newborn to breast as soon as possible.
2. Position baby so that entire body is turned toward breast. Figure 7–1 shows a variety of positions.

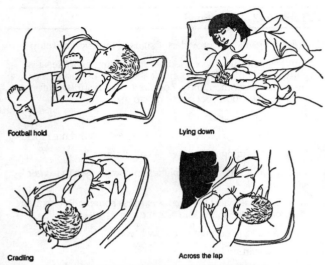

Football hold

Lying down

Cradling

Across the lap

Figure 7–1   Examples of breastfeeding position changes to facilitate thorough breast emptying and prevent nipple soreness.

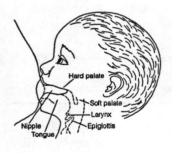

Hard palate

Soft palate

Larynx

Nipple

Tongue

Epiglottis

Figure 7–2   To nurse effectively, it is important that the infant's mouth cover the majority of the areola to compress the ducts below. (Courtesy of Ross Laboratories, Columbus, Ohio.)

3. Direct nipple straight into infant's mouth with as much of the areola included as possible so that as infant sucks, his or her jaws compress the ducts under the areola, where milk is stored (see Figure 7–2).

4. To do this, the mother holds the breast with thumb placed on upper portion and remainder of her fingers cupping the breast. She then lightly strokes the infant's lips with the nipple.

5. Avoid the temptation to use a nipple shield. This confuses the baby and makes it more difficult for him/her to learn to nurse.

6. Avoid setting artificial time limits on the amount of time the baby should nurse. It may take up to three minutes for the letdown reflex to occur. Instead advise the woman to let the baby nurse at one breast as long as he/she is sucking well and positioned correctly. To avoid trauma to the breasts the mother should not let the infant sleep with the nipple in his/her mouth. When the baby has emptied the first breast she/he is burped and switched to the second breast. When the baby has completed feeding she/he is burped again.

7. The baby's suck tends to be most vigorous initially. To avoid undue trauma to the breasts the mother should alternate the breast from which she nurses first.

8. Babies are obligatory nose breathers. To avoid having the breast block the nares, the mother should either lift the breast slightly or compress the breast tissue away from the baby's nose.

Essential Precautions in Practice

During Breastfeeding

Examples of times when disposable gloves should be worn include:

- Assisting the mother to breastfeed the newborn immediately after birth.
- Handling breast milk for breast milk banking.
- Assisting with manual expression of breast milk.
- Handling used breastfeeding pads.

Excellent hand washing is essential when assisting a breastfeeding mother.

REMEMBER to wash your hands prior to putting the disposable gloves on and AGAIN immediately after you remove the gloves.

For further information, consult OSHA and CDC guidelines.

9. To prevent trauma to the nipple the mother should break suction before removing the infant from the breast by inserting a finger into the infant's mouth, next to the nipple.

10. When feeding is completed the woman should wash the nipples with warm water to prevent milk drying and should inspect them for trauma.

11. Frequent nursing helps establish a good supply of milk and prevents nipple trauma from the too vigorous suck of a ravenous infant. Thus, during the first few days the mother should nurse frequently (every 1-1/2 to 3 hours).

12. Table 7–2 cites suggested interventions for common problems.

Bottle Feeding

Bottle feeding is also a nurturing choice for infant feeding and allows both parents to share in this nurturing activity with their child. A variety of commercial formulas are available. Whole milk and skim milk should not be used for children under two years. Whole milk has too high a protein content; skim milk also has too much protein and lacks adequate calories and essential fatty acids.

Bottle feeding technique

1. Formula tends to be digested more slowly, so the bottle-fed infant may go longer between feedings.

2. Infants are usually fed "on demand," which typically is every three to five hours.

3. The mother should assume a comfortable position with adequate arm support so that she can cradle her baby in her arm close to her body.

4. The bottle should be held, not propped, with the baby's head somewhat elevated. Feeding the infant horizontally may result in positional otitis media.

5. The nipple should have a large enough hole to permit milk to flow in drops when the bottle is inverted. Too large an opening may cause overfeeding and regurgitation.

6. The nipple should be pointed directly into the mouth and on top of the tongue. The nipple should be kept full of formula to avoid ingestion of extra air.

7. The infant should be burped at regular intervals, preferably at the middle and end of the feeding, or, during the first few feedings, after about every 1/2 ounce. If the infant was crying vigorously before feeding, he/she should be burped before feeding or after taking just enough formula to calm down.

8. Burping is done by holding the infant upright on the shoulder or by holding the infant in a sitting position on the feeder's lap with the chin and chest supported by one hand. The back is then stroked or patted gently.

9. Newborns frequently regurgitate small amounts. The feeder may find it helpful to keep a "burp cloth" handy. Forceful emesis requires medical evaluation, especially if other symptoms are present.

10. Infants should be encouraged but not forced to feed. Overfeeding can lead to infant obesity.

THE Rh-NEGATIVE MOTHER

A woman who is Rh negative with an indirect Coombs' test negative, and whose infant is Rh positive with a direct Coombs' negative, is given RhIgG (RhoGAM) within 72 hours after childbirth. See Procedure 14: RhIgG Administration, and Drug Guide 9: Rh_o (D) Immune Globulin (Human).

RUBELLA VACCINE

Women who are not immune to rubella (German measles), as evidenced by a titer of less than 1:10, are usually given the rubella vaccine during the immediate postpartal period because it is known that they are not pregnant. Because the rubella vaccine is a live, attenuated vaccine, they are advised **not** to become pregnant for at least 3 to 4 months after receiving it. See Drug Guide 10: Rubella Virus Vaccine.

POSTPARTUM EDUCATION: SELECTED TOPICS

Postpartal Exercises

The woman should be encouraged to begin simple exercises in the hospital and to continue them at home. Exercise helps to improve muscle tone, contributes to postpartum weight loss, and aids in preventing constipation. Many agencies have a booklet on appropriate exercises. Figure 7–3 identifies some commonly used exercises.

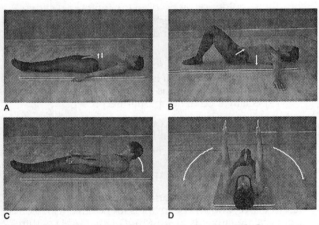

Figure 7–3   Postpartal exercises. Begin with five repetitions two or three times daily and gradually increase to ten repetitions. First day: A, Abdominal breathing. Lying supine, inhale deeply using the abdominal muscles. The abdomen should expand. Then exhale slowly through pursed lips, tightening the abdominal muscles. B, Pelvic rocking. Lying supine with arms at sides, knees bent and feet flat, tighten the abdomen and buttocks and attempt to flatten back on floor. Hold for a count of ten, then arch the back, causing the pelvis to "rock." On the second day add: C, Chin to chest. Lying supine with legs straight, raise head and attempt to touch chin to chest. Slowly lower head. D, Arm raises. Lying supine, arms extended at 90° angle from body, raise arms so they are perpendicular and hands touch. Lower slowly. On fourth day add: E, Knee rolls. Lying supine with knees bent, feet flat, arms extended

Sibling Preparation

Most agencies now permit siblings to visit the postpartum area. This visit reassures the children that their mother is well and still loves them. The parents may ask for advice about dealing with the siblings when mother and baby return from the hospital. The following advice may be helpful:

- If possible, have the father carry the new baby inside so that the mother's arms are free to embrace her other children.

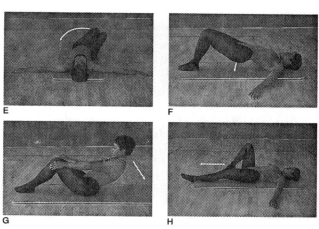

to the side, roll knees slowly to one side, keeping shoulders flat. Return to original position and roll to opposite side. F, Buttocks lift. Lying supine, arms at sides, knees bent, feet flat, slowly raise buttocks and arch the back. Return slowly to the starting position. On the sixth day add: G, Abdominal tighteners. Lying supine, knees bent, feet flat, slowly raise head toward knees. Arms should extend along either side of legs. Return slowly to original position. H, Knee to abdomen. Lying supine, arms at sides, bend one knee and thigh until foot touches buttocks. Straighten leg and lower it slowly. Repeat with other leg. After two to three weeks, more strenuous exercises such as sit-ups and side leg raises may be added as tolerated. Kegel exercises, begun antepartally, should be done many times daily during postpartum to restore vaginal and perineal tone.

- Some mothers bring a doll home for the older sibling. The sibling can then care for the doll when the mother is caring for the baby.
- Involving older children in baby care helps them develop a sense of closeness with the baby. Even very young children can hold the baby with supervision.
- Each parent should spend quality time in a one-to-one experience with each of their older children. Hugs, kisses, and words of praise are also important.
- Regression is common, and a toilet-trained child may begin to wet or may request a bottle for meals.

Resumption of Sexual Activity

The couple is advised to abstain from sexual intercourse until the episiotomy is healed and the lochia has stopped, which is usually by the end of the third week.

- Because the vagina may be dry (hormone-poor), some form of water-soluble lubricant such as K-Y jelly may be necessary to prevent discomfort.
- Warn breastfeeding couples that the woman may leak milk with orgasm because of the release of oxytocin. Some couples find this pleasurable or amusing; others prefer to have the woman wear a bra. Nursing the baby prior to intercourse may help prevent leaking.
- The woman may experience decreased interest in sex due to hormonal changes, fatigue, dissatisfaction with her personal appearance, and lingering discomfort (often related to the episiotomy). This may be frustrating, especially for her partner, and they may find it helpful to discuss the issue openly.
- To avoid an unplanned pregnancy, the couple should be advised to use contraception when they resume sexual activity, even if the woman's menses have not yet returned.

CONTRACEPTION

Contraceptive information should be made available before the woman is discharged. In choosing a method, consistency of use outweighs absolute reliability of a given method. The nurse should review for the woman (or couple) the advantages and disadvantages of each method, risk factors and contraindications, and the ways of using a given method to enable the woman (or couple) to choose the best method for her and her partner. Different methods of contraception may be appropriate at different times in the couple's life. Table 7–3 identifies factors to consider in selecting a method of contraception.

Methods of Contraception

Condom (Male)   A condom is a barrier contraceptive; its effectiveness is increased when it is used in combination with a spermicide.
Advantages: Small, lightweight, disposable, and inexpensive; has no side effects; requires no medical examination or supervision; offers visual evidence of effectiveness; provides some protection against sexually transmitted infections.

Table 7–3   Factors to Consider in Choosing a Method of Contraception

---

Effectiveness of method in preventing pregnancy

Safety of the method:
    Are there inherent risks?
    Does it offer protection against STDs or other conditions?

Client's age and future childbearing plans

Any contraindications in client's health history

Religious or moral factors influencing choice

Personal preferences, biases, etc

Life-style:
    How frequently does client have intercourse?
    Does she have multiple partners?
    Does she have ready access to medical care in the event of complications?
    Is cost a factor?

Partner's support and willingness to cooperate

Personal motivation to use method

Disadvantages: Risk of breakage or displacement; may cause perineal or vaginal irritation, some dulling of sensation.

Method of use: Condoms are applied to the erect penis, rolled from the tip to the end of the shaft before vulvar or vaginal contact is made. A small space is left at the tip to accommodate ejaculate, thereby avoiding breakage. Condom rim should be held when penis is withdrawn from vagina to prevent spillage. Latex may be weakened by prolonged exposure to heat.

Note: Only latex condoms offer protection against AIDS. "Skin condoms" made of lamb's intestine do not.

Condom (Female)   Barrier method; not designed to be used with a male condom.

Advantages: See male condom. Because it covers a portion of the woman's perineum and the base of the penis during intercourse, it may offer increased protection against STDs.

Disadvantages: Higher cost (about $2.25 per condom). Acceptance by couples not yet established.

Method of Use: Thin polyurethane sheath with a flexible ring at each end. Inner ring serves as a means of insertion and covers the cervix like a diaphragm. Second ring remains outside vagina and covers a portion of the perineum. Inner sheath prelubricated. May be inserted up to 8 hours before intercourse. (See Figure 7–4.)

Diaphragm   The diaphragm is a barrier contraceptive used with a spermicidal cream or jelly.

Advantages: Excellent choice for women who are unable or unwilling to take birth control pills or to have an intrauterine device (IUD). Involves no medication; contraception only used as necessary; may be inserted up to four hours before intercourse.

Disadvantages: Women who are not comfortable manipulating their genitals may find it unacceptable; some couples feel it interferes with sexual spontaneity.

Contraindications: A history of toxic shock syndrome or urinary tract infections.

Method of use: A diaphragm must be fitted by a trained care giver. It is inserted into the vagina prior to intercourse with approximately 1 teaspoonful of spermicidal jelly or cream placed around the rim and in the cup. When correctly placed it covers the cervix. If more than

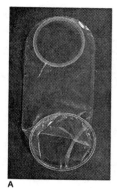

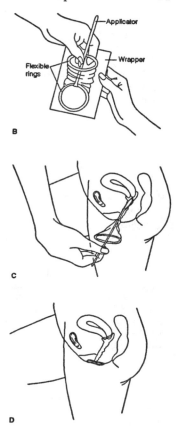

Figure 7–4 **A,** *A female condom. To insert the condom:* **B,** *Remove the condom and applicator from wrapper by pulling up on ring.* **C,** *Insert the condom slowly by gently pushing the applicator toward the small of the back.* **D,** *When the condom is properly inserted, the outer ring should rest on the folds of the skin around the vaginal opening, and the inner ring (closed end) should fit loosely against the cervix.*

4 hours elapse between insertion and intercourse, additional spermicide should be inserted into the vagina (see Figure 7–5). The diaphragm is left in place for at least 6 to 8 hours after intercourse. Then it is removed, cleaned, and allowed to dry. It should be inspected periodically for holes or tears.

Cervical cap   The cervical cap is similar to the diaphragm, except it fits snugly over the cervix. It may be left in place up to 48 hours. Tends to be more difficult for women to insert and remove.

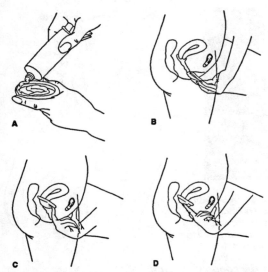

Figure 7–5   Diaphragm and jelly. A, Jelly is applied to the rim and center of the diaphragm. B, Insertion of the diaphragm. C, Rim of the diaphragm is pushed under the symphysis pubis. D, Checking the placement of the diaphragm. Cervix should be felt through the diaphragm.

Fertility Awareness Methods: Also called "natural family planning."
Advantages: Methods are free, safe, acceptable to many whose religious beliefs prohibit other methods; involve no artificial substances or medications; encourage a couple to communicate about sexual activity and family planning; and are useful in helping a family plan a pregnancy.
Disadvantages: Require extensive initial counseling to use effectively; may interfere with sexual spontaneity; require extensive maintenance of records for several cycles prior to beginning use; difficult for women with irregular cycles to use; not as reliable as other methods.
Method of Use: Changes in a woman's cycle (such as changes in mucous, temperature, etc) are used to identify fertile and safe days.

Intrauterine Device (IUD) The IUD provides continuous contraceptive protection by immobilizing sperm and impeding their progress from the cervix through uterus to uterine tubes. May also speed movement of ovum through tubes to uterus. IUD also produces a local inflammatory response. Best suited for multiparous women in a monogamous relationship.

Types available: Copper-containing Cu380T (ParaGard) and progesterone-containing Progestasert.

Advantages: High effectiveness, continuous contraceptive protection, no coitus-related activity, and relative inexpensiveness over time.

Disadvantages: Possible adverse effects including pelvic inflammatory disease (PID), severe dysmenorrhea, irregular menses, increased bleeding during menses, uterine perforation, expulsion; if IUD fails and pregnancy results, there is increased risk of ectopic pregnancy.

Contraindications: History of PID. Not recommended for women with multiple sexual partners because of the increased risk of PID.

Method of use: Requires signed consent before insertion by a physician, nurse midwife, or trained nurse practitioner. The woman should check for the presence of the string once weekly for the first month and then after each menses.

Oral contraceptives Oral contraceptives provide contraceptive protection by inhibiting release of ovum and by maintaining cervical mucus that is hostile to sperm.

Advantages: No coitus-related activity, high effectiveness rate. Noncontraceptive benefits include the following: decreased menstrual cramps, decreased menstrual flow, increased cycle regularity, decreased incidence of functional ovarian cysts. In addition there is a substantial reduction in the incidence of ectopic pregnancy, ovarian cancer, endometrial cancer, iron deficiency anemia, and benign breast disease.

Disadvantages: Must be taken daily; has some serious associated side effects, especially those related to thrombus formation.

Contraindications: Pregnancy, previous history of thrombophlebitis, acute or chronic liver disease, presence of estrogen-dependent carcinoma, undiagnosed uterine bleeding, heavy smoking, hypertension, diabetes, and hyperlipidemia.

Method of use: Pills are prescribed after a careful review of the woman's history and a thorough physical exam including blood pressure (BP) check and Pap smear. The woman is seen yearly while on the pill. Pills are begun on the first Sunday after the beginning of the menstrual cycle and are taken daily for 21 days. The woman then stops for one week (or takes seven "blank" pills if she prefers a 28-day package.) She then resumes the pills. Low-dose pills should be taken within four hours of the same time daily. She should use a backup method such as condoms during her first cycle on the pills. If she misses a pill she should take it when she remembers and take her pill for the day at the regular time. Many women take their pills at night when they are less rushed, so they are asleep when most side effects such as nausea would occur.

Spermicides   Spermicides provide contraceptive protection by destroying sperm or neutralizing vaginal secretions and thereby immobilizing sperm. They are available in a variety of forms including cream, foam, jelly, film, and suppositories. Spermicides are only minimally effective when used alone. Their effectiveness increases when used with a condom.

Advantages: Wide availability and low toxicity. Offers high degree of protection against gonorrhea and some protection against *Chlamydia, Trichomonas,* and herpes.

Disadvantages: Low reliability, some messiness.

Vasectomy   A vasectomy is a male sterilization procedure in which the vas deferens is severed surgically. Relatively simple procedure that does not interfere with erectile function.

Tubal ligation   Tubal ligation is a method of female sterilization in which the uterine tubes are severed. Because it involves general anesthesia, it has more associated risks than a vasectomy.

Both procedures should be considered irreversible despite some success with microsurgical techniques to reverse the operation.

Subdermal implants (Norplant)   Six silastic capsules of levonorgestrel, a progestin, are implanted in the woman's arm. They act by preventing ovulation in most women and by stimulating the production of thick cervical mucus, which inhibits sperm penetration. Requires a minor surgical procedure for insertion.

Advantages: Provides continuous contraception that is removed from the act of coitus. Effects last up to five years.

Disadvantages: Variety of side effects (spotting or irregular bleeding, amenorrhea, weight gain, increased incidence of ovarian cysts, hirsutism, headaches, depression. Implants may be visible in very slender users. Recent literature indicates that the implants are sometimes difficult to remove.

CARE OF THE WOMAN FOLLOWING CESAREAN BIRTH

The new mother who has given birth by cesarean has postpartal needs similar to those of women who give birth vaginally; however, she also has nursing care needs similar to those of women who have undergone major abdominal surgery. Nursing interventions include the following:

1. Encourage woman to cough, deep breathe, and use incentive spirometry every 2 to 4 hours while awake for the first day or two following birth.

2. Encourage leg exercises q2h until woman is ambulatory.

3. Monitor temperature for fever (infection), BP for decrease, and pulse for increase (hemorrhage). Elevated BP may indicate pregnancy-induced hypertension (PIH) (may occur for up to 48 hours postpartum).

4. Assess for adequate voiding after the Foley catheter is removed. Implement nursing interventions if necessary to encourage voiding (privacy, increased fluid, warm water over perineum, ambulation).

5. Assess for evidence of abdominal distention. Note presence or absence of bowel sounds. Measures to prevent or minimize gas pains include leg exercises, abdominal tightening, early ambulation, and avoiding the use of straws. Flatulence may be relieved by lying on the left side, using a rocking chair, and the

use of antiflatulents (such as simethicone), suppositories, and enemas.

6. Measures to alleviate pain include the following:

- Administer analgesics as needed. Patient-
controlled analgesia (PCA) is available in many
facilities.

- Offer comfort through positioning, back rubs,
oral care, and reduction of noxious stimuli such
as noise or odors.

- Encourage presence of significant others, including baby.

- Encourage breathing, relaxation, and distraction
techniques (such as those taught in childbirth
preparation classes).

7. Encourage shower by second postpartal day (cover
incision with plastic wrap until staples are removed,
and stay close in case woman becomes faint).

8. Discharge teaching includes need for adequate rest,
warning signs of infection, ways of lifting and feeding infant to avoid strain.

9. Provide opportunities for parent-infant interaction.

CHAPTER 8

The At-Risk Postpartal Client

POSTPARTAL HEMORRHAGE

Overview

Postpartum hemorrhage is defined as a blood loss of greater than 500 mL at any time after birth. The main causes of postpartal hemorrhage are uterine atony (relaxation of uterus due to hydramnios, large infant, multiple gestation, grand multiparity, use of magnesium sulfate in labor), retained placental fragments, laceration of genital tract, or hematoma development (resulting from trauma to uterus, vagina, or perineum). Postpartum hemorrhage is characterized by bright red vaginal bleeding in the presence of either a soft boggy uterus with clots or a well-contracted uterus without clots. This condition most commonly occurs within the first 24 hours after giving birth. Hematomas present as severe pressure anywhere along the genital tract and purple color to the vaginal mucosa or ecchymotic perineum. Late or delayed hemorrhage occurs after 24 hours after birth, usually within one to two weeks postpartum; except with subinvolution that can occur up to six weeks after birth.

Medical Management

1. **Uterine atony.** Oxytocic drugs are administered after separation of the placenta to prevent uterine atony (see Drug Guide 7: Oxytocin [Pitocin]). Fundal height and firmness are determined; if the uterus is not firm and well contracted after expulsion of the placenta, fundal massage is initiated. 9If there is excessive bleeding (more than 500 mL), the clinician may do bimanual uterine compression.

Oxygen via mask is administered at 6–10 liters per minute. Hematocrit, partial thromboplastin, prothrombin times, and fibrinogen levels are monitored. Methylergonovine maleate (Methergine) IM (see Drug Guide 4) may be ordered for immediate management of uterine atony.

2. **Retained placental fragments.** Inspect the placenta for any signs that a cotyledon or piece of membrane is missing. If missing pieces are suspected the uterine cavity requires uterine exploration. Sonography may be considered to look for retained fragments. Methylergonovine maleate (Methergine) IM or p.o. (see Drug Guide 4) is ordered. Prostaglandins (IM or directly injected into the uterine cavity) may be used for rapid sustained contractions.

3. **Lacerations.** A visual examination of the cervix is made and deep cervical lacerations are sutured to stop the bleeding.

4. **Hematomas.** Small hematomas are managed with ice packs and ongoing observation. They usually reabsorb naturally. Larger hematomas or those increasing in size are incised and drained to achieve hemostasis. Vaginal packing is inserted to achieve hemostasis if needed. Large vaginal packs can make voiding difficult. An indwelling catheter is often necessary. Because incision and drainage may predispose to infection, antibiotics are ordered. Replace blood and clotting factors as needed.

Critical Nursing Assessments

1. Assess BP, pulse, and respirations every 15 minutes × 4, then every 30 × 2 after normal birth. If vaginal bleeding is noted, assess BP, pulse, and respirations q15min.
   Be alert for: Hypotension and tachycardia can be signs of hypovolemia, along with tachypnea, pallor, cyanosis, and cold and clammy skin.

   2. Assess fundal status for height and firmness (see Procedure 8: Fundal Assessment).

Uterus should be firm and at or below the umbilicus. A well-contracted fundus rules out uterine atony.

3. Assess amount of blood loss/vaginal bleeding, any blood clots expressed.
   Assessment technique: Visual assessment, do pad counts within a given time period or weigh the perineal pads (one mL of blood weighs 1 gm).
   Be alert for: To determine the amount of blood loss, assess not only the peripads but also the underpads for pooling of blood. To do so, have the woman turn on her side.

4. Examine perineum and buttocks for discoloration, bulging, tender areas. If woman is still recovering from regional anesthesia, frequent visualization of perineum/buttocks is essential. Palpate obvious masses for tenderness and fluctuation.

5. Examine vagina or rectum for protruding masses.
   Assessment technique: Position woman on her side, raise her upper buttock, and instruct her to bear down.
   Be alert for: Bulging purplish mass may become apparent at the introitus, or a soft mass may be palpable upon rectal exam.

6. Assess for bladder distention (hinders effective uterine contractions and involution process).

7. Assess intake and output q8hrs.
   Be alert for: Urine output needs to stay at > 30 mL/hr to perfuse kidneys well.

8. Assess laboratory results.
   Be alert for: Decreasing hematocrit (500 mL blood loss may be seen as a 4-point decrease in hematocrit) and an increase in prothrombin time or partial thromboplastin time, and a decrease in fibrinogen.

9. Assess woman's coping responses, level of understanding of her condition, and emotional status.

10. Assess woman's ability to take care of her baby because of fatigue related to blood loss. Also assess existing support systems at home.

Sample Nursing Diagnoses

- Fluid volume deficit related to blood loss secondary to uterine atony, retained placental fragments, lacerations, or hematoma formation.
- Risk for infection related to trauma and hemorrhage.
- Risk for injury related to tissue damage secondary to prolonged pressure from a large vaginal hematoma.

Critical Nursing Interventions

1. Gently massage boggy uterus while supporting lower uterine segment (see Figure 8–1) to stimulate contraction and express clots.
   Be alert for: Forceful massage can tire the uterus, resulting in uterine atony, and can cause pain. Be gentle. Don't be misled by the fact that a woman has a firm uterus. Significant bleeding can occur from causes other that uterine atony.

2. Monitor type and amount of bleeding and associated consistency of the uterus.

Essential Precautions in Practice

During Postpartum Hemorrhage

The same basic precautions that apply in caring for any woman during the postpartal period apply when caring for a woman experiencing postpartal hemorrhage. In addition remember the following specifics:

- Wear gloves when assessing the perineum and when changing or disposing of peripads, chux, or linens soiled with blood or body fluids.
- Place blood-soaked disposable material in appropriate waste containers. Store blood-soaked bedding in an appropriate receptacle for the laundry according to agency procedure.
- Wear a splash apron when changing very soiled bedding or helping a clinician control severe hemorrhage.

For further information consult OSHA and CDC guidelines.

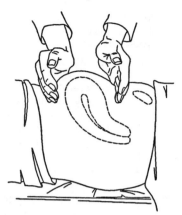

Figure 8–1
Uterine massage.

Be alert for: Dark red blood and relaxed uterus indicate uterine atony or retained placental fragments. Bright red vaginal bleeding and contracted uterus indicate laceration hemorrhage.

3. Monitor vital signs. Note any signs of hypovolemic shock (tachycardia, tachypnea, decreased blood pressure, pallor, oliguria, restlessness, and lethargy).

4. Maintain IV and start second IV with 14-, 16-, or 18-gauge needle to administer blood products if necessary. Send blood for type and cross match if not already done in the birthing area.

5. Administer oxytocics per order. Carefully note uterine tone and blood pressure response to medication.

6. Monitor intake and output hourly. Initially insert Foley catheter to ensure accurate output determination.

7. Provide oxygen via mask or nasal cannula at 7–10 L/min for signs of respiratory distress.

8. Position woman either flat with legs elevated or Trendelenburg per agency protocol to increase blood flow to vital organs.

9. Administer pain medications for discomfort as ordered.

10. Provide stool/chair for use during shower in case of dizziness or weakness to facilitate self-care and progressive ambulation.

11. Review the following critical aspects of the care you have provided:
    - Have I effectively monitored her fundal and lochia status? Did I quickly identify and intervene when there was continued relaxation of the uterus and expression of clots? Did I carry out the uterine massage as gently as possible?
    - Are woman's vital signs stable? Is woman showing any signs of hypovolemia?
    - Is woman complaining of discomfort anywhere along the genital tract? Have I provided adequate comfort measures for her, such as cold/warm packs, perineal care, sitz baths, or pain medication?
    - Have I assisted in decreasing the anxiety of the woman and her family by keeping them informed about her status?
    - Have I provided the mother with home care information, eg, expected changes in fundus and lochia, signs of abnormal bleeding, and when to call health care provider?

Evaluation

Anticipated outcomes of nursing care include:
- Signs of postpartal hemorrhage are detected quickly and managed effectively.
- Hematoma formation is detected quickly and managed successfully.
- The woman's discomfort is relieved effectively.
- The woman is able to identify abnormal changes that might occur following discharge and understands the importance of notifying her care giver if they develop.
- Maternal-infant attachment is maintained successfully

SUBINVOLUTION

Overview

Subinvolution is the failure of the uterus to follow the normal pattern of involution and is one of the most common causes of late postpartum hemorrhage. Primary causes of subinvolution are retained placental fragments or membranes, endometritis, or pelvic infection. Myomas and uterine fibroids are also contributing causes. Usually the signs and symptoms of subinvolution are not apparent until about four to six weeks postpartum. The client, who may not know that her uterus is not involuting properly, may have prolonged blood loss and develop anemia before seeking assistance from a health-care professional.

The fundus remains higher in the abdomen/pelvis than expected. Lochia often fails to progress from rubra to serosa to alba. The lochia may remain rubra or return to rubra several days postpartum. The amount of lochia may be more profuse than expected. Leukorrhea and backache may occur if infection is present. The woman may also relate a history of irregular or excessive bleeding after the birth.

Medical Management

1. **Uterine examination.** Bimanual uterine exam shows an enlarged, softer than normal uterus.

2. **Drug therapy.** Oral methylergonovine 0.2 mg or ergonovine 0.2 mg q3–4 hrs for 24–48 hours is given to stimulate uterine contractility (see Drug Guide 4: Methylergonovine Maleate [Methergine]). Oral antibiotics are ordered if metritis (infection) is present or invasive procedures are done.

3. **Uterine curettage.** If treatment is not effective or if retained placental fragments and polyps are the cause, a dilatation and curettage (D & C) may be done. Polyps can form from fibrotic retained tissues.

Critical Nursing Assessments

1. Assess characteristics of lochial pattern since birth. **Be alert for:** Lochia pattern: Lochia doesn't progress from rubra to serosa or returns to rubra days after the birth.

2. Assess whether mother has felt feverish or has had a temperature.
   Be alert for: Elevation in temperature can occur if infection is cause of subinvolution.

3. Assess woman's level of understanding regarding her condition, the signs of subinvolution, and when she should call her health-care provider.

Sample Nursing Diagnoses

- Pain related to stimulation of uterine contraction secondary to administration of oxytocic medications.
- Risk for infection related to bacterial invasion of uterus secondary to dilatation and curettage.
- Knowledge deficit related to lack of information about delayed postpartum bleeding secondary to failure of normal involution process.

Critical Nursing Interventions

1. During discharge teaching, review normal involution process and progression of lochia from rubra to serosa to alba. Stress that the woman should report any continued bleeding that does not go away with rest and medication and that covers the surface of one perineal pad two to six weeks after birth.

2. Discuss the importance of increasing the length and number of rest periods; see if she can have a support person with her during the 24-hour oxytocic medication period.

3. Review the treatment regimen, the importance of taking medications as directed, and any adverse effects that should be reported to the health-care provider.

4. Inform the lactating woman that she can continue to breastfeed. Low-dose methylergonovine poses no threat to baby, and breastfeeding can assist in involution.

5. If woman has history of elevated blood pressure, teach her the early signs of adverse effects of oxytocic medication on her blood pressure. These include nausea, vomiting, headache, and complaints

of abdominal cramping or signs of circulatory stasis, including itching, tingling, numbness, and cold fingers and toes.

Sample Nurse's Charting

7:30 PM T 99.2F, P 92, R 16, BP 124/76. Fundus soft 1 FB above symphysis pubis and midline. Tender to palpation. Lochia rubra with small clots. Complains of fatigue, lochia flow return to rubra, and soaking surface of one peripad/day 15 days after birth. Is breastfeeding and expresses concern over continued rubra lochia and progressive fatigue. S. Paulski, RNC

Evaluation

- Woman knows the signs of delayed uterine involution and when to report them to her health-care provider.
- Woman understands the treatment regimen and takes her medications as ordered.
- Woman has support to help her deal with increased fatigue and anxiety related to the failure of uterus to return to normal.

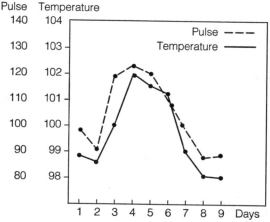

Figure 8–2 *Endometritis vital signs pattern.*

TYPES OF REPRODUCTIVE TRACT INFECTIONS

Type/Cause	Signs/Symptoms	Treatment
Localized Infection of External Genitals Episiotomy or sutured laceration; infected traumatized perineum, vulva, vagina, or abdominal incision	Low-grade fever (< 38.3C [101F]), localized pain, edema, redness, seropurulent discharge Late: skin discoloration, shock, wound abscess, high temperature and chills	Oral antibiotics and antibiotic creams, removal of stitches to promote drainage, use of gauze to keep lesion open, sitz baths, analgesics
Endometritis (Metritis) Infection of total endrometrium or placental site	Sawtooth fever pattern (low grade to 103F [39.4C] see Figure 8–2), chills, rapid pulse. Headache, backache, malaise, loss of appetite, cramps. Large, boggy, tender uterus. Scant to profuse dark brown, foul-smelling discharge. In βhemolytic infection, scant and odorless lochia.	IV antibiotics (cephalosporin or ampicillin), oxytocics to stimulate contraction and lochial drainage, semi-Fowler's position and/or ambulation to promote drainage (aerobic and anaerobic), blood and lochial culture, D & C for retained placental tissue, hydration (oral/IV)
Parametritis (Pelvic Cellulitis) Infection of tissues around uterus via the lymphatics (often following endometritis)	Prolonged high fever (102–104F, [38.9-40C]), chills, abdominal tenderness on one or both sides. Pain when uterus is moved during pelvic exam. Vaginal, rectal, abdominal abscesses	Broad spectrum antibiotics (IV/PO). Hydration (up to 2000 mL/day), blood transfusion for decreasing hemoglobin, bed rest, analgesics

Critical Nursing Assessments

1. Assess BP, pulse, and respirations every two to four hours. Tachycardia is associated with endometritis.

2. Assess temperature every four hours unless elevated, then q2hr. **Tip:** Remember that a low-grade fever is common during the first 24 hours after birth. Be alert for elevated temperature (greater than 100.4F [38C]) patterns.

3. Assess fundal height, tone, and sensation (see Procedure 8: Fundal Assessment). Note any discomfort or pain that is greater than anticipated, and note protracted afterpains.

4. Assess perineum every eight hours. Inspect perineum using good light source. **Assessment technique:** Have woman lie on her side with her top leg slightly forward and ahead of the bottom leg (see Figure 8–3). After donning disposable gloves, lift the buttock to expose the perineum and the anus. If no episiotomy is present the perineum is described as "intact." Assess episiotomy or sutured laceration for redness, edema, ecchymosis, discharge, approximation of edges (skin edges together) and tenderness (REEDA scale).

5. Assess lochia for type, amount, and odor (see Procedure 4: Evaluation of Lochia after Birth).

6. Assess laboratory results for above normal postpartum levels, especially the white blood cell count. **Tip:** Normal postpartum leukocyte levels are already increased (15,000–30,000/mm^3) so be alert for > 30,000/mm^3.

7. Assess hydration status.

8. Assess for abscess formation (often a palpable mass and fever).

Sample Nursing Diagnoses

- Risk for infection related to broken skin or traumatized tissues.

- Knowledge deficit related to lack of information about reproductive tract infections and their treatment.

- Altered parenting related to mother's malaise and other symptoms of infection.

Critical Nursing Interventions

1. Monitor temperature every four hours and identify trends.
   Be alert for: Low-grade fever (< 101F [38.3C]) with rapid onset indicates localized infection. Irregular fever (sawtooth pattern), varying from 101–103F (38.3–39.4C) indicates endometritis. Persistent high fever (102–104F [38.9–40C]) and chills indicate parametritis.

2. Monitor lochial changes for signs of failure of normal involution.

3. Teach woman about, and perform, proper perineal and hygienic measures to promote healing and prevent contamination of the perineum, such as washing hands frequently and after each peripad change, perineal care (see Chapter 7), and use of sitz baths or surgigator. Encourage a diet high in protein and vitamin C.

4. Obtain cultures of lochia, wound, and urine (to rule out asymptomatic urinary tract infection).
   Tip: With episiotomy infections, lochia may have a foul odor and appear yellow.

5. Administer antibiotics, oxytocics (see Drug Guide 7: Oxytocin [Pitocin], and Drug Guide 4: Methylergonovine Maleate [Methergine]), and analgesic spray as prescribed. Instruct on need to take entire course of prescribed medications at home.

6. Assist mothers with endometritis to ambulate and lie in semi-Fowler's position to facilitate lochial drainage.

7. If parametritis occurs, provide bed rest and maintain IV fluids. Monitor intake and output and urine specific gravity.

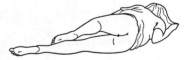

Figure 8–3   Episiotomy is inspected. Woman is on her side, and her upper leg is forward.

8. Teach woman with draining wound or purulent lochia about wound care and proper management of soiled dressings and linen.

9. Institute home care referral as needed.

10. Maintain mother-infant interaction. Assist mother to balance her need for rest and her need for time with her baby.

Evaluation

- The infection is quickly identified and treated successfully without further complications.

- The woman understands the infection and the purpose of therapy; she carries out any ongoing antibiotic therapy if indicated following discharge.

- Maternal-infant attachment is maintained.

THROMBOEMBOLIC DISEASE

Overview

Thromboembolic disease refers primarily to superficial thrombophlebitis (thrombus due to inflammation), which primarily forms in saphenous veins, appears on third or fourth postpartal day, and shows clinical improvement within 48 hours of therapy. Thrombophlebitis often presents as a slight temperature elevation over the area of vein inflammation, mild calf pain, visible and palpable veins, and possibly a positive Homans' sign. Deep vein thrombosis is seen in women with a history of thrombosis and increases the likelihood of pulmonary emboli development. Deep vein thrombosis may present with severe leg pain of sudden onset (pain may worsen if leg is in a dependent position and if pressure is applied to calf area), edema and paleness of affected leg, systemic signs of elevated temperature, pulse and chills, and possible positive Homans' signs. Deep vein thrombosis may take up to four to six weeks to resolve after the acute symptoms stop.

Medical Management

1. **Superficial thrombophlebitis.** Bed rest with leg elevation is ordered. Moist heat therapy is applied to facilitate drainage and decrease venous stasis. Elastic support hose are to be worn after acute inflammation subsides.

2. **Deep vein thrombosis.** In addition to treatment for superficial thrombophlebitis, anticoagulant therapy is ordered. Heparin via continuous IV of 1 unit/mL of estimated blood volume or subcutaneous 5000 to 7500 units q4–6hrs is ordered dependent on the results of activated partial thromboplastin time (APTT). The desired APTT lab value is 1-1/2–2-1/2 X control in seconds. No aspirin or ibuprofen can be taken by women on anticoagulant therapy.

   Special alert: One-percent protamine sulfate is used as the antidote for anticoagulant overdose.

Critical Nursing Assessments

1. Assess vital signs, especially oral temperature q4hrs. Be alert for and report temperature > 100.4F.

2. Assess calves, thighs, and groin area (especially left side) bilaterally for increase in size, color, warmth, peripheral pulses, and positive Homans' sign. **Assessment technique for Homans' sign:** Dorsiflex foot with knee in extended position (see Figure 8–4). If pain occurs in foot or leg with foot dorsiflexion, Homans' sign is positive.

3. Assess CBC, platelet count, prothrombin time, and partial prothrombin time results.

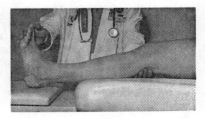

Figure 8–4 Homans' sign: With the woman's knee flexed to decrease the risk of embolization, the nurse dorsiflexes the foot. Pain in the foot or leg is a positive Homans' sign.

4. Assess for evidence of bleeding related to heparin therapy.

Sample Nursing Diagnoses

- Altered peripheral tissue perfusion related to venous stasis.
- Altered tissue perfusion related to pulmonary embolism secondary to dislodgement of deep vein thrombus.

Critical Nursing Interventions

1. Monitor vital signs.
   Be alert for: elevated temperature, which may be associated with inflammation.

2. Inspect and palpate calf, thigh, and groin area daily for heat, color, tenderness, and peripheral pulses.
   Be alert for: increasing redness, swelling, or pain.

3. Monitor any signs of deep vein thrombosis.
   Be alert for: sudden onset of severe leg or thigh pain, elevated temperature, or chills. Report these signs to physician immediately.

4. Measure affected portion of leg with nonstretch tape to assess degree of edema.

5. Assist mother to stay on bed rest with her leg fully elevated on pillows. Do not use knee gatch on bed and avoid any pressure on popliteal space (to prevent pelvic pooling and impedance of blood flow). While mother is on bed rest, have her use footboard, do passive exercises, and change position frequently.

6. Apply warm packs to affected leg (vasodilatation facilitates blood flow and decreases pain). Be sure to wrap packs to prevent burns and remove for ten minutes each hour.

7. Administer antibiotics per order.

8. Administer heparin as ordered after obtaining APTT results. Monitor APTT and Hct to evaluate bleeding and adequacy of heparinization. Have 1% protamine sulfate on hand for heparin overdose.

9. Initiate progressive ambulation after acute inflammation subsides.

10. Apply support hose (compresses superficial veins and increases deep venous flow).

11. Monitor and report signs of pulmonary emboli. **Be alert for:** signs such as vague chest pain, anxiety, respiratory rate > 16 breaths/minute, pallor, tachypnea, and possible changes in lung sounds (rales and friction rub).

12. Instruct mother on measures to prevent venous stasis:

    - Avoid crossing legs at the knee while sitting.
    - Elevate the feet while sitting when possible.
    - Avoid prolonged standing.
    - Ambulate periodically throughout the day.
    - Drink at least six 8-oz. glasses of water/day.

13. Instruct mother regarding anticoagulant therapy:

    - Take medication at the same time each day.
    - Keep appointments so that clotting times can be monitored and medication can be adjusted.
    - Maintain current eating habits (include green vegetables) and life-style.
    - Avoid any activities that may cause bleeding, such as playing contact sports, using stiff toothbrushes, or shaving legs with a straight razor.
    - Be aware of signs of heparin overdose such as bleeding gums, ecchymosis, nosebleed, hematuria, and melena.
    - Note any blood in the stools; it should be reported to the physician.
    - Wear a Medic-Alert bracelet indicating use of anticoagulants.
    - Avoid medications such as aspirin and non-steriodal anti-inflammatory drugs that increase anticoagulant activity.

14. If woman wishes to continue breastfeeding, have her discuss use of low-dose subcutaneous heparin at home rather that warfarin.

15. Review the following critical aspects of the care you have provided:

    - Have I administered the correct dose of heparin at the designated times after first reviewing the APTT results?

    - Have I been alert for any signs of heparin overdose?

    - What can I do to assist the woman to maintain bed rest?

    - Is mother able to eat a diet that assists her coagulation status?

    - Have I assessed the woman's understanding of her thrombolic status and answered her questions? Have I given her opportunities to practice preventive measures?

16. Review with the couple the signs and symptoms of thrombophlebitis and the need to report them since it may not occur until after discharge.
    Be alert for: Do not massage affected leg.

Evaluation

- If thrombosis/thrombophlebitis develops, it is detected quickly and managed successfully without further complications.

- At discharge the woman is able to explain the purpose, dosage regimen, and necessary precautions associated with any prescribed medications such as anticoagulants.

- The woman can discuss self-care measures and on-going therapies (such as the use of elastic stockings) that are indicated.

- The woman has bonded successfully with her newborn and is able to care for the baby effectively.

MASTITIS

Overview

Mastitis refers to an inflammation of the breast commonly caused by *Staphylococcus aureus* from the infant's nose and throat. Contributing factors include clogged milk ducts, bruised tissue, unclean hands, and cracked or fissured nipples. *Candida albicans* is another cause of mastitis. Mastitis usually occurs in the 2nd or 4th week postpartum. A breast abscess may be a complication.

Medical Management

1. **Drug therapy.** Antibiotics are ordered for a full ten-day course even if symptoms subside within a few days. Antipyretics such as acetaminophen are used.

2. **Breastfeeding.** Breastfeeding is stopped only in the presence of large amounts of nipple drainage. In the presence of a yeast infection, the mother and baby are both treated with nystatin for 14 days.

3. **Laboratory tests.** Infectious mastitis is usually indicated by elevated leukocyte and bacterial counts.

4. **Breast abscess management.** If a breast abscess forms, the breast milk and any drainage is cultured. The abscessed area is incised, drained, and packed with sterile gauze.

Critical Nursing Assessments

1. Examine breast for localized redness, tenderness, and swelling. On palpation, it may be very hard and hot and the lump may feel like a hard "moth ball."

2. Inspect nipple for fissures or cracks (entry points for infection).
   Be alert for: If nipples are inflamed and painful consider a yeast or fungus infection. Breast abscesses appear as hardened, painful local areas of inflammation below the skin surface.

3. Assess mother's general physical status. Systemic symptoms include flulike symptoms: headache, malaise, muscle ache, rapid pulse, and temperature about 38.5C (101.3F).

4. Assess mother's dietary and sleep patterns, and level of stress. Decreases in diet and sleep and/or exces-

sive stress and activity can decrease mother's resistance to infection.

5. Assess feeding history for precipitating factors such as ineffective emptying of breasts, engorgement, breast compression from tight clothing or bra, or sudden change in feeding pattern such as baby sleeping through the night or use of supplemental feedings.

6. Inspect baby's mouth for white patches surrounded by redness on the buccal membrane, which indicate *Candida albicans,* or thrush.

Sample Nursing Diagnoses

- Pain related to development of mastitis.
- Knowledge deficit related to lack of information about appropriate breastfeeding practices.
- Risk for infection related to cracked and traumatized breast tissue or nipples.
- Ineffective breastfeeding related to interrupted breastfeeding schedule.

Critical Nursing Interventions

Preventive measures

1. Discuss predisposing factors.

2. Use good hand washing technique.

3. Instruct mother about breast care: hand washing before handling breasts or nipples, cleansing of breast with water only (to maintain protective oils), wearing supportive bra at all times (to avoid milk stasis in lower lobes), changing bra and breast pads frequently.

4. Reinforce mother's knowledge about breastfeeding techniques, such as position, frequency, removal of baby from breast.

5. Provide special attention to mothers who have blocked milk ducts, which increase the risk for mastitis.

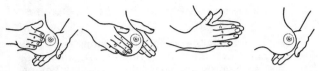

Figure 8–5 Breast massage. Caked areas of breast are massaged toward the nipple.

If the woman has mastitis

1. Administer medications as ordered. Oral pain medications are given 20 minutes before feeding to ease discomfort.

2. Teach mother to increase feeding frequency, increase fluid intake (six to eight 8-oz glasses a day), have friends or relatives assist with care in order to increase rest periods, breastfeed first on unaffected breast until letdown occurs (promotes complete emptying of both breasts), express milk at least every three hours, and massage caked areas toward nipple during feeding (see Figure 8–5).

3. Mother's temperature should be monitored every four hours until infection resolves.

4. Instruct mother that if there is no improvement within 12–14 hours or if fever persists, she should notify her health care provider. If mother is on antibiotics and the baby develops diarrhea, she should let her physician know.

5. Provide support if mother needs to discontinue breastfeeding temporarily and instruct her on expression of milk (see Procedure 13: Methods of Breast Pumping and Milk Storage).

Evaluation

- The mother is able to identify predisposing factors, signs and symptoms of impending mastitis, and preventive measures.

- Mother knows proper management if mastitis should occur. Mother is supported in her decision to breastfeed and knows how to resume if it is necessary to stop.

URINARY TRACT INFECTION

Overview

Most postpartal urinary tract infections (UTIs) are caused by gram-negative organisms such as *Escherichia coli,* which invade the urethra and bladder and cause cystitis. Postpartal women are at increased risk because of decreased bladder sensitivity due to stretching, trauma, and retention of residual urine; bacteria introduced during catheterization; and bladder trauma during childbirth. Bladder bacteria then may ascend to the kidney as a result of vesicoureteral reflux during voiding, causing pyelonephritis. Clinical signs may not appear for several days. The woman may then present with dysuria, urinary urgency and frequency, suprapubic or lower abdominal pain, lower back discomfort, and possibly hematuria. In addition to the signs and symptoms of cystitis, pyelonephritis presents as cloudy urine and systemic signs of high fever, chills, nausea and vomiting (N & V), malaise, fatigue, severe flank pain, and costovertebral angle tenderness (CVAT). Cystitis management must continue after symptoms disappear, since this infection tends to recur.

Medical Management

1. **Urinalysis.** Urinalysis is obtained and analyzed for protein, blood, and organisms. Urine that contains an increase in WBCs, (>100,000/mL organisms or too numerous to count) and protein and/or blood indicates UTI. Urine culture and sensitivities are obtained so organism-specific antibiotics can be identified. Urine cultures are obtained one week after therapy is completed and at four to six week intervals for at least a year to monitor for recurring infections.

2. **Fluid and drug management.** Fluid intake is increased to three to four L/day to dilute the urine and initiate flushing out of the infected urine. Therapeutic doses of vitamin C or cranberry juice are used to acidify the urine. Urine acidification decreases bacterial growth and increases the action of urinary tract antiseptics. Short-acting sulfonamides such as sulfisoxazole (Gantrisin) are ordered for ten days

except in term pregnancy, when sulfamethoxazole/
trimethoprim (Septra, Bactrim) may be given.
Urinary tract antiseptics (Azo Gantrisin) or systemic
antibiotics (ampicillin or cephalosporins qid for
7–10 days) can also be used.

3. **Pyelonephritis management.** If woman develops
pyelonephritis, she may be hospitalized for aggres-
sive treatment and monitoring to prevent permanent
kidney damage. Intravenous medications are given
and an indwelling bladder catheter may be put in
place. Relief of symptoms is usually obtained in 24
to 48 hours.

Critical Nursing Assessments

1. Assess bladder function for frequency, urgency,
   and amount of urine output. Inspect urine for color
   (hematuria), odor, appearance (concentrated
   or dilute).

2. Palpate for large mass, at or near umbilicus, that
   displaces uterine fundus upward, denoting an
   overdistended bladder.

3. Assess for painful or burning urination.

4. Assess for complaints of suprapubic or lower
   abdominal discomfort or lower back pain, severe
   flank pain.

5. Palpate for costovertebral tenderness.

6. Assess vital signs q4hrs and observe for signs of
   systemic involvement.

7. Assess intake and output q8hrs.

Sample Nursing Diagnoses

- Altered patterns of urinary elimination related to
  urinary tract infection.
- Risk for injury related to urinary stasis secondary to
  overdistention.
- Knowledge deficit related to lack of information
  about urinary tract infection, its treatment, and possible sequelae.

Critical Nursing Interventions

1. Take vital signs and monitor for fever.

2. Obtain clean-catch, midstream sample for urinalysis.

3. Encourage woman to void q2–3hrs and empty bladder completely. Provide ice pack for perineum within one hour after birth to decrease edema formation and facilitate voiding.

4. If taking cranberry juice, woman should drink at least 240 mL a day.

5. Provide comfort measures such as back massage and analgesics for back and flank pain; anti-spasmodics for dysuria and cramping, antiemetics for N & V, and oral hygiene to promote comfort. If woman has a fever provide tepid baths and antipyretics.

6. If woman is taking sulfonamide drugs, instruct her that breastfeeding should be discontinued and teach her how to pump her breasts (see Procedure 13: Methods of Breast Pumping and Milk Storage). **Be alert for:** Sulfonamides are secreted in breast milk and combine with proteins to create neonatal jaundice; therefore, pumped milk should be discarded while mother is on these medications.

7. Monitor baby for diarrhea and yeast infections (candidiasis) while mother is taking ampicillin.

8. Instruct mother that her urine may change color with prescribed medication. **Be alert for:** Azo Gantrisin can turn urine red or red orange; nitrofurantoin creates brown urine, may cause N & V and diarrhea, and should be taken with food or milk to decrease gastric irritation.

9. Reinforce instruction on prophylactic hygienic practice, eg, wiping from front to back, voiding when she feels the urge to void, wearing cotton underclothing, and voiding after intercourse. Encourage woman to drink two glasses of water immediately after intercourse in order to increase urine output and flush out contaminants that may have entered the urethra.

Evaluation

- Woman understands any special instructions for taking medications and need for follow-up urine culture.
- Woman knows hygienic, nutritional, and fluid requirements to avoid urinary tract infections and any symptoms to report to health care provider.

ONGOING MANAGEMENT OF SELECTED PERINATAL COMPLICATIONS

Pregnancy-Induced Hypertension (PIH)

The postpartum goal is to prevent eclamptic seizures and neurologic sequelae.

Effect of postpartum on PIH	Critical Nursing Interventions
Postpartum diuresis decreases serum magnesium sulfate levels, thereby increasing the possibility of seizures.	Monitor vital signs (VS) closely for 48 hours after birth (vital signs should remain stable then begin to slowly decrease). Monitor urine output (< 30 mL/hr) and deep tendon reflexes (DTRs).
	Administer IV magnesium sulfate for 24 hours after birth.
	Check urine for protein and specific gravity qhr.
	Administer diuretic as ordered. Do not give oxytocics because of their hypertensive properties.
	Minimize environmental stimuli until status improves.
	Have seizure precautions in place.
Magnesium sulfate causes uterine relaxation, which increases the possibility of uterine atony; PIH decreases blood volume and lowers platelet counts, which can lead to postpartum hemorrhage.	Monitor for signs of postpartum hemorrhage. Carefully massaging the uterus is important.
	Encourage frequent voiding to keep bladder empty and avoid uterine atony.
	Emotional support is essential during critical illnesses.

Diabetes

The goal is to maintain normal blood glucose levels, prevention of postpartum complications (PIH, hemorrhage, infection) and enhance parent-infant interaction.

Effect of Postpartum on Diabetes

Critical Nursing Interventions

Loss of placental insulin inhibitory hormone (human chorionic somatomammotrophin [hCS], progesterone) drops insulin requirement sharply. Some women do not require insulin for the first day or so.

Draw blood glucose immediately after birth. Monitor urine for glucose and ketones q2hr x 24 hours. Administer insulin on sliding scale based on blood or urine glucose test per physician order.

Increased use of glucose during postpartum.

Monitor for hypoglycemia (see Chapter 2). Maintain IV glucose for 24 hours after birth then restart diabetic diet.

Increased postpartum complications, such as PIH.

Monitor VS for at least 48 hours. Be alert for PIH symptoms (see Chapter 2).

Hemorrhage due to uterine atony and increased amniotic fluid.

Monitor uterine involution.

Any infection complicates diabetic regulation and increases risk of acidosis.

Maintain excellent hand washing for self. Stress personal hygiene to avoid infections.

Altered parent-infant interaction because baby requires special observation.

Promote flexible visiting policy.

Keep parents informed of baby's progress and status.

If mother is breastfeeding have her increase her caloric intake by 400–500 kcal/day (20% protein); adjust insulin dosage as needed per physician order. Provide for pumping or breastfeeding opportunities q2–4 hours around the clock.

Betamethasone
(Celestone® Soluspan®)

Overview of Maternal-Fetal Action

Studies have provided ample evidence that glucocorticoids such as betamethasone are capable of inducing pulmonary maturation and decreasing the incidence of respiratory distress syndrome in preterm infants. The mechanism by which corticosteroids accelerate fetal lung maturity is unclear, but it is related to the stimulation of enzyme activity by the drug. The enzyme is required for biosynthesis of surfactant by the type II pneumocytes. Surfactant is of major importance to the proper functioning of the lung in that it decreases the surface tension of the alveoli. Glucocorticoids also increase the rate of glycogen depletion, which leads to thinning of the interalveolar septa and increases the size of the alveoli. The thinning of the epithelium brings the capillaries into closer proximity with the air spaces and improves oxygen exchange (Blackburn & Loper 1992). Black female newborns have shown the largest decrease in respiratory distress syndrome after this therapy; White males have been much less responsive (Williams 1991). Only the first-born twin appears to benefit from antenatal steroid therapy (Briggs et al 1994).

Route, Dosage, Frequency

Prenatal maternal intramuscular injections of 12 mg of betamethasone are given once a day for 2 days. Dexamethasone may also be given in doses of 6 mg every 12 hours for four doses (NIH Consensus Development Conference 1994). To obtain maximum results, birth should be delayed for at least 24 hours after completing the first round of treatment. The effect of corticosteroids may be transient. Currently, it is suggested that the treatment regime be repeated every week up to 34 weeks' gestation for the undelivered fetus with an immature lung profile.

Contraindications

Inability to delay birth for 24 to 48 hours

Adequate L/S ratio

Presence of a condition that necessitates immediate birth (eg, maternal bleeding)

Presence of maternal infection, diabetes mellitus, hypertension

Gestational age greater than 34 completed weeks

Maternal Side Effects

Bishop (1981) reports that suspected maternal risks include (1) initiation of lactation, (2) increased risk of infection, (3) augmentation of placental insufficiency in hypertensive women, (4) gastrointestinal bleeding, (5) inability to use estriol levels to assess fetal status, (6) possible pulmonary edema when used concurrently with tocolytics (such as ritodrine).

May cause Na^+ retention, K^+ loss, weight gain, edema, indigestion.

May mask signs and symptoms of infection.

Effects of Fetus/Neonate

Lowered cortisol levels at birth but rebounds within 2 hrs of age (Briggs et al 1994).

Hypoglycemia.

Increased risk of neonatal sepsis (Briggs et al 1994).

Animal studies have shown serious fetal side effects such as reduced head circumference, reduced weight of the fetal adrenal and thymus glands, and decreased placental weight (Briggs et al 1994). Human studies have not shown these effects, however.

Nursing Considerations

Assess for presence of contraindications.

Provide education regarding possible side effects.

Administer betamethasone deep into gluteal muscle, avoiding injection into deltoid (high incidence of local atrophy). (Dexamethasone may be administered IM or IV.)

Periodically evaluate BP, pulse, weight, and edema.

Assess lab data for electrolytes and blood glucose.

Although concomitant use of betamethasone and toco-lytic agents has been implicated in increased risk of pul-monary edema, betamethasone has little mineral corticoid activity; therefore, it probably doesn't add significantly to the salt and water retention effects of beta-adrenergic agonists. Other causes of noncardiogenic pulmonary edema should also be investigated if pulmonary edema develops during administration of betamethasone to a woman in preterm labor.

Erythromycin (Ilotycin) Ophthalmic Ointment

Overview of Neonatal Action

Erythromycin (Ilotycin) is used as prophylactic treatment of ophthalmia neonatorum, which is caused by the bac-teria *Neisseria gonorrhoeae*. Preventive treatment of gon-orrhea in the newborn is required by law. Erythromycin is also effective against ophthalmic chlamydial infections. It is either bacteriostatic or bactericidal depending on the organisms involved and the concentration of drug.

Route, Dosage, Frequency

Ophthalmic ointment (0.5%) is instilled as a narrow rib-bon or strand, 1/4-inch long, along the lower conjunctival surface of each eye, starting at the inner canthus. It is in-stilled only once in each eye. Administration may be done in the birthing area or later in the nursery so that eye con-tact is facilitated and the bonding process immediately after birth is not interrupted. After administration, gently close eye and manipulate to ensure spread of ointment.

Neonatal Side Effects

Sensitivity reaction; may interfere with ability to focus and may cause edema and inflammation. Side effects usually disappear in 24–48 hours.

Nursing Considerations

Wash hands immediately prior to instillation to prevent introduction of bacteria.

Do not irrigate the eyes after instillation. Use new tube or single-use container for ophthalmic ointment administration shortly after birth. May wipe away excess after 1 minute.

Observe for hypersensitivity.

Teach parents about need for eye prophylaxis. Educate them regarding side effects and signs that need to be reported to the health care provider.

Magnesium Sulfate (MgSO₄)

Pregnancy Risk Category: B

Overview of Obstetric Action

$MgSO_4$ acts as a CNS depressant by decreasing the quantity of acetylcholine released by motor nerve impulses and thereby blocking neuromuscular transmission. This action reduces the possibility of convulsion. For this reason, $MgSO_4$ is used in the treatment of preeclampsia. Because magnesium sulfate secondarily relaxes smooth muscle, it may decrease the blood pressure, although it is not considered an antihypertensive. $MgSO_4$ may also decrease the frequency and intensity of uterine contractions; as a result it is also used as a tocolytic in the treatment of preterm labor.

Route, Dosage, Frequency

$MgSO_4$ is generally given intravenously to control dosage more accurately and prevent overdosage. Some physicians still prescribe intramuscular administration. However, IM administration is painful and irritating to the tissues and does not permit the close control that IV administration does.

The intravenous route allows for immediate onset of action. It must be given by infusion pump for accurate dosage.

For Treatment of Preterm Labor

Loading dose: 6 g $MgSO_4$ 250 mL solution is administered over a 30 minute period (Parsons & Spellacy 1994).

Maintenance dose: 2–4 g/hour via infusion pump (Parsons & Spellacy 1994).

For Treatment of Preeclampsia

Loading dose: 4–6 g $MgSO_4$ as a 20% solution is administered over a 15–20 minute period (Arias 1993).

Maintenance dose: 1–2 g/hour via infusion pump (Mandeville & Troiano 1992).

Note: $MgSO_4$ is excreted via the kidneys. Because women in preterm labor typically have normal renal function, they generally require higher levels of magnesium to achieve a therapeutic range than women who have preeclampsia and may have compromised renal function (Parsons & Spellacy 1994).

Maternal Contraindications

Diagnosed maternal myasthenia gravis is the only absolute contraindication to the administration of $MgSO_4$ (Mandeville & Troiano 1992). A history of myocardial damage or heart block is a relative contraindication to use of the drug because of the effects on nerve transmission and muscle contractility. Extreme care is necessary in administration to women with impaired renal function because the drug is eliminated by the kidneys, and toxic magnesium levels may develop quickly.

Maternal Side Effects

Most maternal side effects are dose related. Lethargy and weakness related to neuromuscular blockade are common. Sweating, a feeling of warmth, flushing, and nasal congestion may be related to peripheral vasodilation. Other common side effects include nausea and vomiting, constipation, visual blurring, headache, and slurred speech. Signs of developing toxicity include depression or absence of reflexes, oliguria, confusion, respiratory depression, circulatory collapse, and respiratory paralysis. Rapid administration of large doses may cause cardiac arrest.

Effects on Fetus/Neonate

The drug readily crosses the placenta. Some authorities suggest that transient decrease in FHR variability may occur; others report that no change occurred. In general $MgSO_4$ therapy does not pose a risk to the fetus. Long-term therapy may result in fetal hypocalcemia (Briggs et al 1994). Occasionally, the newborn may demonstrate neurologic depression or respiratory depression, loss of reflexes, and muscle weakness (Briggs et al 1994). Ill effects in the newborn may actually be related to fetal growth retardation, prematurity, or perinatal asphyxia (Knuppel & Drukker 1993). Toxicity is not usually correlated with cord serum magnesium levels. Observe newborn closely for first 24–48 hours after birth.

Nursing Considerations

1. Monitor the blood pressure closely during administration.

2. Monitor maternal serum magnesium levels as ordered (usually every 6–8 hours). Therapeutic levels are in the range of 4–8 mg/dL. Reflexes often disappear at serum magnesium levels of 8–10 mg/dL; respiratory depression occurs at levels of 10–15 mg/dL; cardiac conduction problems occur at levels above 15 mg/dL (Scott 1994).

3. Monitor respirations closely. If the rate is less than 12/minute, magnesium toxicity may be developing, and further assessments are indicated. Many protocols require stopping the medication if the respiratory rate falls below 12/minute.

4. Assess knee jerk (patellar tendon reflex) for evidence of diminished or absent reflexes. Loss of reflexes is often the first sign of developing toxicity (Sibai 1990). Also note marked lethargy or decreased level of consciousness and hypotension.

5. Determine urinary output. Output less than 30 mL/hour may result in the accumulation of toxic levels of magnesium.

6. If the respirations or urinary output fall below specified levels or if the reflexes are diminished or

absent, no further magnesium should be administered until these factors return to normal.

7. The antagonist of magnesium sulfate is calcium. Consequently, an ampule of calcium gluconate should be available at the bedside. The usual dose is 1 gm given IV over a period of about 3 minutes.

8. Monitor fetal heart tones continuously with IV administration.

9. Continue $MgSO_4$ infusion for approximately 24 hours after birth as prophylaxis against postpartum seizures if given for PIH.

10. If the mother has received $MgSO_4$ close to birth, the newborn should be closely observed for signs of magnesium toxicity for 24–48 hours.

Note: Protocols for magnesium sulfate administration may vary somewhat according to agency policy. Consequently individuals are referred to their own agency protocols for specific guidelines.

Methylergonovine Maleate (Methergine)

Overview of Obstetric Action

Methylergonovine maleate is an ergot alkaloid that stimulates smooth muscle tissue. Because the smooth muscle of the uterus is especially sensitive to this drug, it is used postpartally to stimulate the uterus to contract in order to decrease blood loss by clamping off uterine blood vessels and to promote the involution process. In addition, the drug has a vasoconstrictive effect on all blood vessels, especially the larger arteries. This may result in hypertension, particularly in a woman whose blood pressure is already elevated.

Route, Dosage, and Frequency

Methergine has a rapid onset of action and may be given intramuscularly, orally, or intravenously.

Usual IM dose: 0.2 mg following delivery of the placenta. The dose may be repeated every 2–4 hours if necessary.

Usual oral dose: 0.2 mg every 4 hours (six doses).

Usual IV dose: Because the adverse effects of Methergine are far more severe with IV administration, this route is seldom used.

Maternal Contraindications

Pregnancy, hepatic or renal disease, cardiac disease, and hypertension contraindicate this drug's use.

Maternal Side Effects

Hypertension (particularly when administered IV), nausea, vomiting, headache, bradycardia, dizziness, tinnitus, abdominal cramps, palpitations, dyspnea, chest pain, and allergic reactions may be noted.

Effects on Fetus/Neonate

Because Methergine has a long duration of action and can thus produce tetanic contractions, it **should never be used during pregnancy or in labor,** when it may result in fetal trauma or death.

Nursing Considerations

1. Monitor fundal height and consistency and the amount and character of the lochia.

2. Assess the blood pressure before and routinely throughout drug administration.

3. Observe for adverse effects or symptoms of ergot toxicity.

Postpartum Epidural Morphine

Overview of Obstetric Action

Epidural morphine is used to provide relief of pain associated with cesarean birth, extensive episiotomies (mediolaterals), or third- and fourth-degree lacerations. Epidural morphine pain relief results directly from its effect on the opiate receptors in the spinal cord (it depresses pain impulse transmission). Morphine binds opiate receptors, thereby altering both the perception of and emotional response to pain. Women experience little or no discomfort or pain during recovery and for up to 24 hours afterward. There is no motor or sympathetic block or associated hypotension. Onset of analgesia is slower, but duration is longer.

Route, Dosage, Frequency

Five to seven and one-half mg of morphine is injected through a catheter into the epidural space, providing pain relief for about 24 hours.

Maternal Contraindications

Allergy to morphine, narcotic addiction, or chronic debilitating respiratory disease.

Maternal Side Effects

Late onset respiratory depression (rare but may occur 8–12 hours after administration), nausea and vomiting (occurring between four and seven hours after injection), itching (begins within three hours and lasts up to ten hours), urinary retention, and, rarely, somnolence. Side effects can be managed with naloxone.

Neonatal Effects

No adverse effects since medication is injected after birth of baby.

Nursing Considerations

Assess client's sensitivity to narcotics on admission.

Monitor and evaluate analgesic effect. Ask client about comfort level and notify anesthesiologist of inadequate pain relief.

Check catheter for obvious knots, breaks, and leakage at insertion site and catheter hub.

Assess for pruritus (scratching and rubbing, especially around face and neck).

Naloxone Hydrochloride (Narcan)

Overview of Neonatal Action

Naloxone hydrochloride (Narcan) is used to reverse respiratory depression due to acute narcotic toxicity. It displaces morphine-like drugs from receptor sites on the neurons; therefore, the narcotics can no longer exert their depressive effects. Naloxone reverses narcotic-induced respiratory depression, analgesia, sedation; hypotension, and pupillary constriction.

Route, Dosage, Frequency

Intravenous dose is 0.1 to 0.2 mg/kg of 1.0 mg/mL or 0.25 mL/kg of 0.4 mg/mL concentration at birth, including premature infants. This drug is usually given through the umbilical vein or endotracheal tube, although naloxone can be given intramuscularly or subcutaneously. The use of neonatal naloxone (Narcan 0.02 mg/mL) is no longer recommended by the American Academy of Pediatrics Committee on Drugs because of the extremely small fluid volumes.

Reversal of drug depression occurs within 1 to 2 minutes. The duration of action is variable (minutes to hours) and depends on the amount of the drug present and rate of excretion. Dose may be repeated in 5 minutes. If there is no improvement after two or three doses, discontinue naloxone administration. If initial reversal occurs, repeat dose as needed.

Neonatal Contraindications

Should not be administered to infants of narcotic-addicted mothers because it may precipitate acute withdrawal syndrome.

Respiratory depression resulting from nonmorphine drugs such as sedatives, hypnotics, anesthetics, or other nonnarcotic CNS depressants.

Neonatal Side Effects

Excessive doses may result in irritability, increased crying, and prolongation of partial thromboplastin time (PTT).

Tachycardia.

Nursing Considerations

Monitor respirations closely—rate and depth.

Assess for return of respiratory depression when naloxone effects wear off and effects of longer-acting narcotics reappear.

Have resuscitative equipment, O_2, and ventilatory equipment available.

Monitor bleeding studies.

Note that naloxone is incompatible with alkaline solutions.

Oxytocin (Pitocin)

Overview of Obstetric Action

Oxytocin (Pitocin) exerts a selective stimulatory effect on the smooth muscle of the uterus and blood vessels. Oxytocin affects the myometrial cells of the uterus by increasing the excitability of the muscle cell, increasing the strength of the muscle contraction, and supporting propagation of the contraction (movement of the contraction from one myometrial cell to the next). Its effect on the uterine contraction depends on the dosage used and on the excitability of the myometrial cells. During the first half of gestation little excitability of the myometrium occurs, and the uterus is fairly resistant to the effects of oxytocin. However, from midgestation on, the uterus responds increasingly to exogenous intravenous oxytocin. Cautious use of diluted oxytocin, administered intravenously at term results in a slow rise of uterine activity.

The circulatory half-life of oxytocin is 3–5 minutes. It takes approximately 40 minutes for a particular dose of oxytocin to reach a steady-state plasma concentration (Arias 1993).

The effects of oxytocin on the cardiovascular system can be pronounced. There may be an initial decrease in the blood pressure, but with prolonged administration, a 30% increase in the baseline blood pressure may be noted. Cardiac output and stroke volume are increased. With doses of 20 mU/minute or above, the antidiuretic effect of oxytocin results in a decrease of free water exchange in the kidney and a marked decrease in urine output (Marshall 1985).

Oxytocin is used to **induce** labor at term and to **augment** uterine contractions in the first and second stages of labor. Oxytocin may also be used **immediately after birth to stimulate uterine contraction** and thereby control uterine atony.

Route, Dosage, Frequency

For induction of labor: Add 10 units Pitocin (1 mL) to 1000 mL of intravenous solution. (The resulting concentration is 10 mU oxytocin per 1 mL of intravenous fluid.) Using an infusion pump, administer IV, starting at 0.5–1 mU/min and increase by 1–2 mU/minute every 40–60 minutes. Or start at 1–2 mU/minute and increase by 1 mU/minute every 15 minutes until a good contraction pattern (every 2–3 minutes and lasting 40–60 seconds) is achieved.

Maternal Contraindications

Severe preeclampsia-eclampsia (PIH)

Predisposition to uterine rupture (in nullipara over 35 years of age, multigravida 4 or more, overdistention of the uterus, previous major surgery of the cervix or uterus)

Cephalopelvic disproportion

Malpresentation or malposition of the fetus, cord prolapse

Preterm infant

Rigid, unripe cervix; total placenta previa

Presence of fetal distress

Maternal Side Effects

Hyperstimulation of the uterus results in hypercontractility, which in turn may cause the following:

Abruptio placentae

Impaired uterine blood flow → fetal hypoxia

Rapid labor → cervical lacerations

Rapid labor and birth → lacerations of cervix, vagina, perineum, uterine atony, fetal trauma

Uterine rupture

Water intoxication (nausea, vomiting, hypotension, tachycardia, cardiac arrhythmia) if oxytocin is given in electrolyte-free solution or at a rate exceeding 20 mU/minute; hypotension with rapid IV bolus administration postpartum.

Effect on Fetus/Neonate

Fetal effects are primarily associated with the presence of hypercontractility of the maternal uterus. Hypercontractility causes a decrease in the oxygen supply to the fetus, which is reflected by irregularities and/or decrease in FHR.

Hyperbilirubinemia (Arias 1993).

Trauma from rapid birth.

Nursing Considerations

Explain induction or augmentation procedure to client.

Apply fetal monitor and obtain 15- to 20-minute tracing and NST to assess FHR before starting IV oxytocin.

For induction or augmentation of labor, start with primary IV and piggyback secondary IV with oxytocin and infusion pump.

Ensure continuous fetal and uterine contraction monitoring.

The maximum rate is 40 mU/minute (ACOG 1988). Not all protocols recommend a maximum dose. When indicated, it is generally between 16 and 40 mU/minute (Owen & Hauth 1992). Decrease oxytocin by similar increments once labor has progressed to 5–6 cm dilatation (ACOG 1988; Arias 1993).

0.5 mU/min = 3 mL/hr	8 mU/min = 48 mL/hr
1.0 mU/min = 6 mL/hr	10 mU/min = 60 mL/hr
1.5 mU/min = 9 mL/hr	12 mU/min = 72 mL/hr
2 mU/min = 12 mL/hr	15 mU/min = 90 mL/hr
4 mU/min = 24 mL/hr	18 mU/min = 108 mL/hr
6 mU/min = 36 mL/hr	20 mU/min = 120 mL/hr

Protocols may vary from one agency to another.

Assess FHR, maternal blood pressure; pulse; and uterine contraction frequency, duration, and resting tone before each increase in oxytocin infusion rate.

Record all assessments and IV rate on monitor strip and on client's chart.

Record oxytocin infusion rate in mU/minute and mL/hour (eg, 0.5 mU/minute [3 mL/hr]).

Record all client activities (such as change of position, vomiting), procedures done (amniotomy, sterile vaginal examination), and administration of analgesics on monitor strip to allow for interpretation and evaluation of tracing.

Assess cervical dilatation as needed.

Apply nursing comfort measures.

Discontinue IV oxytocin infusion and infuse primary solution when (1) fetal distress is noted (bradycardia, late or variable decelerations; (2) uterine contractions are more frequent than every 2 minutes; (3) duration of contractions exceeds more than 60 seconds; or (4) insufficient relaxation of the uterus between contractions or a steady increase in resting tone are noted (ACOG 1988). In addition to discontinuing IV oxytocin infusion, turn client to side, and if fetal distress is present, administer oxygen by tight face mask at 6–10 L/minute. Notify physician.

Maintain intake and output record.

For augmentation of labor:

Prepare and administer IV Pitocin as for labor induction. Increase rate until labor contractions are of good quality. The flow rate is gradually increased at no less than every 30 minutes to a maximum of 10 mU/minute (Cunningham et al 1993). In some settings or in a situation when limited fluids may be administered, a more concentrated solution may be used. When 10 U Pitocin is added to 500 mL IV solution, the resulting concentration is 1 mU/minute = 3 mL/hour. If 10 U Pitocin is added to 250 mL IV solution, the concentration is 1 mU/minute = 1.5 mL/hr.

For administration after delivery of placenta:

One dose of 10 units Pitocin (1 mL) is given intramuscularly or by slow intravenous push or added to IV fluids for continuous infusion.

Assess FHR, maternal blood pressure, pulse, and uterine contraction frequency, duration, and resting tone before each increase in oxytocin infusion rate.

Record all assessments and IV rate on monitor strip and on client's chart. Record oxytocin infusion rate in mU/minute and mL/hour (eg, 0.5 mU/minute [3 mL/hr]).

Record all client activities (such as change of position, vomiting), procedures done (amniotomy, sterile vaginal examination), and administration of analgesics on monitor strip to allow for interpretation and evaluation of tracing.

Assess cervical dilatation as needed.

Apply nursing comfort measures.

Discontinue IV oxytocin infusion and infuse primary solution when (1) fetal distress is noted (tachycardia or bradycardia, late or variable decelerations), (2) uterine contractions are more frequent than every 2 minutes, (3) duration of contractions exceeds 60 seconds, or (4) insufficient relaxation of the uterus between contractions or a steady increase in resting tone are noted (ACOG 1988). In addition to discontinuing IV oxytocin infusion, turn client to side, and if fetal distress is present, administer oxygen by tight face mask at 6–10 L/minute; notify physician.

Maintain intake and output record. Asses intake and output every hour.

Recombinant Hepatitis B Vaccines

Overview of Neonatal Action

Recombinant hepatitis B vaccines are used as a prophylactic treatment against all subtypes of hepatitis B virus. The vaccine provides passive immunization for newborns of HBsAg-negative and HBsAg-positive mothers. Hepatitis B can be transmitted across the placenta, but most newborns are infected during birth. The vaccines are produced from bakers' yeast and plasmid containing the HBsAg gene.

Hepatitis B vaccine contains more that 95% HBsAg protein and is an inactivated (noninfective) product. Universal immunization is recommended.

Infants of HBsAg-positive mothers should concurrently receive 0.5 mL of hepatitis B immunoglobulin (HBIG) prophylaxis.

Route, Dosage, Frequency

The first dose of 0.5 mL (10 μg) is given intramuscularly into the anterolateral thigh within 12 hours of birth for infants born to HBsAg-positive mothers. The second dose of vaccine is given at 1 month of age and followed by a final dose at 6 months of age.

Infants born to HBsAg-negative mothers receive their first dose of vaccine at birth, the second dose at 1–2 months, and the third dose at 6–18 months (American Academy of Pediatrics 1992).

Infants whose mother's HBsAg status is unknown receive the same doses as infants born to HBsAg-positive mothers.

Neonatal Side Effects

The only common side effect is soreness at the injection site. Occasionally, there is erythema, swelling, warmth, and induration at the injection site or a low-grade fever.

Nursing Considerations

Delay administration during active infection; the vaccine will not prevent infection during its incubation period.

The vaccine should be used as supplied. Do not dilute.

Do not inject intravenously or interdermally.

Monitor for adverse reactions. Monitor temperature closely.

Have epinephrine available to treat possible allergic reactions.

Responsiveness to the vaccine is age dependent. Preterm infants weighing less than 1000 gm have lower seroconversion rates. Consider delaying the first dose until the infant is term PCA (postconceptual age) or use a four-dose schedule.

Rh$_o$ (D) Immune Globulin (Human) (RhoGAM, Gamulin Rh, HypRho-D, MICRhoGAM, Mini-Gamulin RH)

Overview of Obstetrical Action

Rh$_o$ (D) immune globulin is a concentrated solution of immunoglobulin (IgG) that contains anti-Rh$_o$ (D) from human fractionated plasma. It functions by suppressing the immune response of nonsensitized Rh$_o$ (D)-negative women who are exposed to Rh$_o$ (D or D^u) positive blood. It prevents maternal isoimmunization by lysis of fetal Rh-positive red blood cells (RBCs) that may be circulating in the maternal blood stream after birth. RhoGAM prevents hemolytic disease of the newborn. In addition, it is given to Rh-negative women exposed to Rh-positive blood after abortion, miscarriage, and amniocentesis.

Route, Dosage, Frequency

IM injection in deltoid. Single-dose vials. One standard dose (300 μg) vial given for antepartum prophylaxis at approximately 28 weeks to Rh-negative woman unless father of the baby is known to be Rh-negative, for Rh-negative unimmunized woman undergoing amniocentesis, and for postpartum prophylaxis within 72 hours of birth if lab tests indicate no sensitization has occurred. Multiple dose is required when fetomaternal hemorrhage is > 30 mL. Microdose preparation (50 μg) is given to unsensitized Rh-negative woman who aborts before 13 weeks.

Maternal Contraindications

Previous sensitization, hypersensitization, Rh$_o$ (O)-positive/D^u-positive client.

Maternal Side Effects

Irritation at injection site, fever, lethargy, and myalgia. Potential allergic reaction, rare systemic reactions.

Nursing Considerations

Note the blood type and Rh status of all pregnant women.

Send Rh blood workup on mother and baby and cord blood for type and cross match on baby.

If large fetomaternal transfusion is suspected, it may be necessary to send blood for Betke-Kleihauer or D^u test, which detect 20 mL or more of Rh-positive fetal blood in the maternal circulation.

Confirm that the following criteria for administration are present: Mother must be Rh negative with no Rh antibodies present (negative indirect Coombs' test) in order to receive Rh immune globulin.

Client teaching: Instruct Rh-negative woman that the drug needs to be given after subsequent births if the baby is Rh positive. She should carry information on Rh status and dates of RhoGAM injections with her at all times.

Check preparation with another nurse. Ensure correct vial is used for the client (each vial is cross matched to the specific woman and must be carefully checked).

Administer IM only in deltoid; inject entire contents of vial, and aspirate prior to injecting.

Assess for tenderness at injection site and any other side effects.

Do not administer discolored/precipitated solutions.

Keep solutions stored in refrigerator.

Record lot number, route, dose, client education, and any other data per agency policy.

Rubella Virus Vaccine (Meruvax 2)

Overview of Obstetrical Action

Rubella vaccine is a live attenuated virus that stimulates active immunity against the rubella virus. Rubella acquired during pregnancy may result in congenital rubella syndrome (CRS), with associated fetal anomalies. The greatest risk period for the fetus is from one week prior to four weeks after conception. Women who have not had rubella or who are serologically negative (ie, titer of 1:10 or less) are candidates for the vaccination to prevent fetal anomalies in future pregnancies. It should be given in the immediate postpartum period and/or if avoidance of pregnancy for at least three months can be assured. Nursing mothers can be vaccinated since live, attenuated rubella virus is neither communicable nor excreted in breast milk. If mother receives both rubella vaccine and RhoGAM, antibody formation to rubella may be suppressed by the RhoGAM injection.

Route, Dosage, Frequency

Single-dose vial; inject subcutaneously in outer aspect of the upper arm (deltoid).

Maternal Contraindications

Women with allergies to ducks or duck eggs (may have a hypersensitivity reaction and require adrenalin), women with allergy to neomycin (vaccine contains neomycin), women on immunosuppression drugs (corticosteroids, irradiation, alkylating agents, or antimetabolites), or women who have received a blood transfusion, plasma transfusion, or serum immune globulin within the previous three months. If pregnancy status is unknown, do not give vaccine, as it may be teratogenic.

Maternal Side Effects

Burning or stinging at the injection site. Two to four weeks later, a transient rash over the body, arthralgia, malaise, sore throat, or headache may occur.

Nursing Considerations

Instruct women to **avoid pregnancy for three months** following vaccination.

Provide information on contraceptives and their use.

Check if woman has signed an informed consent form (per agency protocol) and received written information about the vaccine, its side effects, and risks.

Ascertain whether mother is to receive RhoGAM as well as rubella and instruct mother that a rubella titer should be redrawn in about three months.

Sodium Bicarbonate

Overview of Neonatal Action

Sodium bicarbonate is an alkalizing agent. It buffers an increase in hydrogen ions caused by accumulation of lactic acid from anaerobic metabolism occurring during hypoxemia. Sodium bicarbonate thereby raises the blood pH, reversing the metabolic acidosis. Sodium bicarbonate should be used to correct severe metabolic acidosis in asphyxiated newborns only once adequate ventilation has been established.

Note: Sodium bicarbonate dissociates in solution into sodium ion and carbonic acid, which can split into water and carbon dioxide. The carbon dioxide must be eliminated via the respiratory tract.

Route, Dosage, Frequency

For resuscitation and severe asphyxiation: intravenous slow push via umbilical vein catheter (infuse at rate no faster than 1 mEq/kg/minute). Dosage is 2 mEq/kg: 4 mL of 0.5 mEq/mL (4.2%) or 2 mL of 1 mEq/mL (8.4%). An 8.4% solution diluted at least 1:1 with sterile water to decrease the osmolarity. Can repeat every 15 minutes if needed for total of four doses. For marked metabolic acidosis: a pH of less than 7.05 and a base deficit of 15 mEq/L or more should be corrected using a 0.5 mEq/mL solution of sodium bicarbonate at a rate of 1 mEq/kg/minute or slower. Calculate total dosage by the following formula:

$$mEq = 0.3 \times weight\ (kg) \times base\ deficit\ in\ mEq/L$$

Neonatal Contraindications

Inadequate respiratory ventilation that causes a rise in P_{CO_2} and a decrease in pH

Presence of edema; metabolic or respiratory alkalosis; and hypocalcemia, anuria, or oliguria

Neonatal Side Effects

Hypernatremia, hyperosmolarity, fluid overload

Intracranial hemorrhage (rapid infusion of bicarbonate increases serum osmolarity, causing a shift of interstitial fluid into the blood and capillary rupture)

Nursing Considerations

Assess for any contraindications.

Monitor intake and output rates.

Assess adequacy of ventilation by monitoring respiratory status, rate, and depth; ventilate as necessary.

Dilute bicarbonate prior to administration into umbilical vein catheter (for resuscitation) or peripheral IV to prevent sloughing of tissue.

Evaluate effectiveness of drug by monitoring arterial blood gases for P_{CO_2}, bicarbonate concentration, and pH determination.

Incompatible with acidic solutions.

Administration with calcium creates precipitates

Vitamin K_1 Phytonadione (AquaMEPHYTON)

Overview of Neonatal Action

Phytonadione is used in prophylaxis and treatment of hemorrhagic disease of the newborn. It promotes liver formation of the clotting factors II, VII, IX, and X. At birth the neonate does not have the bacteria in the colon that is necessary for synthesizing fat-soluble vitamin K_1, therefore the newborn may have decreased levels of prothrombin during the first 5–8 days of life reflected by a prolongation of prothrombin time.

Route, Dosage, Frequency

Intramuscular injection is given in the vastus lateralis thigh muscle. A one-time only prophylactic dose of 0.5–1 mg IM is given in the birthing area or upon admission to the newborn nursery. A one-time dose of 2 mg is given if the route of administration is by mouth. If the mother received anticoagulants during pregnancy, an additional dose may be ordered by the physician and is given at 6–8 hours post first injection (Briggs et al 1994).

Neonatal Side Effects

Pain and edema may occur at injection site. Possible allergic reactions such as rash and urticaria.

Nursing Considerations

Observe for bleeding (usually occurs on second or third day). Bleeding may be seen as generalized ecchymoses or bleeding from umbilical cord, circumcision site, nose, or gastrointestinal tract. Results of serial PT and PTT should be assessed.

Observe for jaundice and kernicterus, especially in preterm infants.

Observe for signs of local inflammation.

Protect drug from light.

Give vitamin K_1 before circumcision procedure.

Administer comfort measures for narcotic-induced pruritus, such as: lotion, back rubs, cool/warm packs, or diversional activities. If the itching can be tolerated, naloxone should be avoided, especially since it counteracts the pain relief.

If allergic reaction (urticaria, edema, or respiratory difficulties) occurs, administer naloxone or diphenhydramine per physician order.

Provide comfort measures for nausea/vomiting, such as frequent oral hygiene or gradual increase of activity; administer naloxone, and antiemetics per physician order.

Assess postural blood pressure and heart rate before ambulation.

Assist client with her first ambulation and then as needed.

Assess respiratory function every hour for 24 hours, then q2–8 hrs as needed. Also assess level of consciousness and mucous membrane color. May need to monitor client via apnea monitor for 24 hours.

Monitor urinary output and assess bladder for distention. Assist client to void.

REFERENCES

American College of Obstetricians and Gynecologists: *Induction and Augmentation of Labor.* Technical Bulletin No. 110 Washington, DC, 1988.

American Academy of Pediatrics: *Guidelines for Perinatal Care,* 3d ed. Chicago: American Academy of Pediatrics, 1992.

Arias F: *Practical Guide to High-Risk Pregnancy and Delivery,* 2d ed. St. Louis: Mosby-Yearbook, 1993.

Bishop EH: Acceleration of fetal pulmonary maturity. *Obstet Gynecol* 1981;58(Suppl):48.

Blackburn ST, Loper DL: *Maternal, Fetal, and Neonatal Physiology: A Clinical Perspective.* Philadelphia: Saunders, 1992.

Briggs GG, Freeman RK, Yaffe SJ: *Drugs in Pregnancy and Lactation,* 4th ed. Baltimore: Williams & Wilkins, 1994.

Cunningham FG, MacDonald PC, Gant NF (eds): *Williams Obstetrics,* 19th ed. Norwalk, CT: Appleton & Lange, 1993.

Knuppel RA, Drukker JE: Hypertension in pregnancy. In: *High-Risk Pregnancy: A Team Approach,* 2d ed. Knuppel RA, Drukker JE (eds). Philadelphia: Saunders, 1993.

Mandeville L, Troiano N: *High-Risk Intrapartum Nursing.* Philadelphia: Lippincott, 1992.

Marshall C: The art of induction/augmentation of labor. *J Obstet Gynecol Neonat Nurs.* January/February 1985;14:22.

National Institute of Health Consensus Development Conference: Effect of corticosteroids for fetal maturation on perinatal outcomes. In: *Yearbook of Neonatal and Perinatal Medicine–1994,* Fanaroff AA, Klaus MH (eds). St. Louis: Mosby, 1994.

Owen J, Hauth JC: Oxytocin for the induction or augmentation of labor. *Clin Obstet Gynecol. 1992;35(3):464.*

Parsons MT, Spellacy WN: Causes and management of preterm labor. In: *Danforth's Obstetrics and Gynecology,* 7th ed. Scott JR et al (eds). Philadelphia: Lippincott, 1994.

Scott JR: Hypertensive disorders of pregnancy. In: *Danforth's Obstetrics and Gynecology,* 7th ed. Scott JR et al (eds). Philadelphia: Lippincott, 1994.

Sibai BM: Preeclampsia-eclampsia: Valid treatment approaches. *Contemp Obstet Gynecol.* August 1990;35:84.

Williams MC: Preterm labor. In: *Manual of Obstetrics: Diagnosis and Therapy.* Niswander KR, Evans AT (eds). Boston: Little, Brown, 1991.

Amniocentesis: Nursing Responsibilities

Nursing Action	Rationale
Objective: Prepare woman.	
Explain procedure.	
Reassure woman.	Information will decrease anxiety.
Have woman sign consent form.	Signing indicates woman's awareness of risks and consent to procedure. It is the physician's responsibility to obtain informed consent.
Have woman empty bladder.	Emptying bladder decreases risk of bladder perforation when amniocentesis is done in 3rd trimester.
Objective: Prepare equipment.	
Collect supplies:	
22-gauge spinal needle with stylet	
10-mL syringe	
20-mL syringe	
Three 10-mL test tubes with tops (amber-colored or covered with tape)	Amniotic fluid must be shielded from light to prevent breakdown of bilirubin.

(continued)

Amniocentesis: Nursing Responsibilities *(continued)*

Nursing Action	Rationale
Objective: Monitor vital signs.	
Obtain baseline data on maternal BP, pulse, respiration, and FHR.	Status of woman and fetus is assessed.
Monitor every 15 minutes.	
Objective: Locate fetus and placenta.	
Assist with real-time ultrasound to assess needle presentation during the procedure.	Real-time ultrasound is used to identify fetal parts and placenta and locate pockets of amniotic fluid. Amniocentesis is usually performed laterally in the area of fetal small parts where pockets of amniotic fluid are usually seen.
Objective: Cleanse abdomen.	
Prep abdomen with cleansing agent.	Incidence of infection is decreased.
Objective: Collect specimen of amniotic fluid. (See Essential Precautions in Practice during Amniocentesis.)	
Obtain test tubes from physician; provide correct identification; send to lab with appropriate lab slips.	
Objective: Reassess vital signs.	
Determine woman's BP, pulse, respirations, and FHR; palpate fundus to assess fetal and uterine activity;	Fetus may have been inadvertently punctured. Uterine contractions may ensue following procedure; treatment course

monitor woman with external fetal monitor for 20–30 minutes after amniocentesis.

Have woman rest on left side.

Assess blood type and need for RhoGAM.

Objective: Complete client record.

Record type of procedure done, date, time, name of physician performing test, maternal-fetal response, and disposition of specimen.

Objective: Educate woman.

Reassure woman; instruct her to report any of the following side effects to her primary care taker:

1. Unusual fetal hyperactivity or lack of movement
2. Vaginal discharge—clear drainage or bleeding
3. Uterine contractions or abdominal pain
4. Fever or chills

5. Encourage light activity for 24 hours.

6. Encourage increased oral fluids.

---

should be determined to counteract any supine hypotension and to increase venous return and cardiac output.

Client records will be complete and current.

Client will know how to recognize side effects or conditions that warrant further treatment.

Decrease in maternal activity will decrease uterine irritability and increase uteroplacental circulation.

Increased hydration will replace the amniotic fluid through uteroplacental circulation.

Assessment for Amniotic Fluid

Nursing Action	Rationale
Objective: Assemble equipment.	
Gather Nitrazine test tape and a pair of disposable gloves.	Nitrazine test tape reacts to alkaline fluids and confirms presence of amniotic fluid.
May need microscope and glass slide if determining ferning of obtained fluid.	Microscope is used to detect ferning pattern.
Objective: Set the stage for the assessment.	
Explain the procedure, indications for the procedure, and information that may be obtained. Determine whether she has noted the escape of any clear fluid from the vagina.	Explanation of the procedure decreases anxiety and increases relaxation.
Objective: Test fluid.	
Prior to doing a vaginal exam that uses lubricant, put on gloves. With one gloved hand, spread the labia, and with the other hand place a small section (approx. 2 inches long) against the vaginal opening. You may also place the test tape against any clothing or pads that have been	Contamination of the Nitrazine test tape with lubricant can make the test unreliable.

Enough fluid needs to be placed on the test tape to make it wet. Amniotic fluid is alkaline, and an alkaline fluid |

soaked with possible amniotic fluid. Take care not to touch tape with bare fingers prior to the test.

Compare the color on the test tape to the guide on the back of the Nitrazine test tape container to determine the test results.

turns the Nitrazine test tape a dark blue. If the test tape remains a beige color, the test is negative for amniotic fluid.

Amniotic fluid may also be obtained by speculum exam. Some labor and birth nurses are using this technique. If fluid is present in sufficient amount to draw some into a syringe, a small amount of fluid can be placed on a glass slide, allowed to dry, and then looked at under a microscope. A ferning pattern confirms the presence of amniotic fluid.

Obtaining a specimen by speculum exam reduces the contamination of the fluid with other substances such as blood.

Objective: Record information on client's record.

Record on labor record, eg, SROM, Nitrazine positive

Nurse documents status of membranes, intact or ruptured.

Deep Tendon Reflexes and Clonus Assessment

Nursing Action	Rationale
Objective: Assemble and prepare equipment.	
Obtain a percussion hammer. If one is not available, the side of the hand is also useful in assessing DTRs.	A percussion hammer permits accurate delivery of a brisk tap.
Objective: Prepare woman.	
Explain the procedure, indications for the procedure, and information that will be obtained. At a minimum the patellar reflex should be checked. Most nurses check a second reflex such as the biceps, triceps, or brachioradialis.	Explanation decreases anxiety and increases cooperation. Deep tendon reflexes (DTRs) are assessed to gain information about CNS status and to assess the effects of $MgSO_4$ if the woman is receiving it.
Objective: Elicit reflexes.	
Biceps reflex. The woman's arm is flexed at the elbow with the nurse's thumb placed on the biceps tendon. The nurse's thumb is struck in a slightly downward motion and response is assessed. Normal response is flexion of the arm.	Correct positioning and technique is essential to elicit the reflex. The correct position causes the muscle to be slightly stretched. Then when the tendon is stretched with the tap, the muscle should contract.
Patellar reflex. The woman is positioned with her legs hanging over the edge of the bed (feet should not be	

(continued)

touching the floor). She may also lie supine with her knees slightly flexed and supported by the nurse. The nurse briskly strikes the patellar tendon, which is located just below the patella. Normal response is extension or a thrusting forward of the foot.

Objective: Grade reflexes.

Reflexes are graded on a scale of 1+ to 4+ . See the following table.

Deep Tendon Reflex Rating Scale

Rating	Assessment
4+	Hyperactive; very brisk, jerky, or clonic response; abnormal
3+	Brisker than average; may not be abnormal
2+	Average response; normal
1+	Diminished response; low normal
0	No response; abnormal

Normally reflexes are 1+ or 2+. With CNS irritation hyperreflexia may be present; with high magnesium levels reflexes may be diminished or absent.

Deep Tendon Reflexes and Clonus Assessment (*continued*)

Nursing Action	Rationale
Objective: Assess for clonus.	
With the knee flexed and the leg supported, vigorously dorsiflex the foot, maintain the dorsiflexion momentarily and then release.	Clonus indicates more pronounced hyperreflexia and is indicative of CNS irritability.
Normal response: The foot returns to its normal position of plantar flexion. Clonus is present if the foot "jerks" or taps against the examiner's hand. If so, the number of taps or beats of clonus is recorded.	
Objective: Report and record findings.	
For example: DTRs 2+, no clonus or DTRs 4+, 2 beats clonus.	Provides a permanent record.

Evaluation of Lochia after Birth

Nursing Action	Rationale
Objective: Prepare woman.	
Explain the procedure, the reason for carrying out the procedure, and information that will be obtained.	Explanation of procedure decreases anxiety and increases relaxation.
Objective: Obtain and evaluate maternal vital signs.	
Assess maternal temperature, blood pressure, and pulse.	Provides information regarding physiologic status.
Objective: Accurately evaluate the amount of lochia after birth.	
Put on disposable gloves prior to the assessment.	To observe universal precautions and avoid contact with body substances.
Lower perineal pad so that amount of lochia can be visualized.	Allows nurse to view amount of lochia collected during the assessment.
Palpate uterine fundus by placing one hand on the fundus and the other hand just over the symphysis pubis and press downward. With the other hand, palpate the uterine fundus.	The fundus is located in the midline at the umbilicus or 1 to 2 fingerbreadths below the umbilicus.

(continued)

Evaluation of Lochia after Birth (*continued*)

Nursing Action	Rationale
Determine firmness of fundus.	Downward pressure exerted just above the symphysis pubis prevents excessive downward movement of the uterus during assessment.
	The uterus needs to remain firmly contracted to prevent excessive blood loss.
If fundus is boggy, massage by rubbing in circular motion.	Manual pressure stimulates uterine contractions.
Evaluate the color and amount of lochia, and observe for the presence of clots. The following guidelines may be used to evaluate and describe the amount of lochia: Small: smaller than a 4-in. stain on the pad; 10 to 25 mL Moderate: smaller than a 6-in. stain; 25 to 50 mL Large: larger than 6-in. stain; 50 to 80 mL (Luegenbiehl et al 1990)	Provides information regarding expected status. After birth, a moderate amount of lochia rubra, without clots, is expected.
If blood loss exceeds above guidelines, the perineal pads and the chux may be weighed to estimate blood loss more accurately.	An estimate may be obtained by using the equivalent of 1 gm of weight equals 1 mL. Weighing the pads and chux can provide important information, as amounts of blood loss may be underestimated because of the expectation that some blood will be lost normally.

Exchange Transfusion: Nursing Responsibilities*

Nursing Action	Rationale
Objective: Prepare infant.	
1. Keep newborn NPO for four hr preceding exchange transfusion or aspirate stomach.	To decrease chance of regurgitation and aspiration by neonate.
2. May administer salt-poor albumin (1 g/kg body weight) one hr before exchange transfusion.	To increase binding of bilirubin. Do not give to severely anemic or edemic neonate or to neonate with congestive heart failure, because of hazard of hypervolemia.
3. Assess vital signs.	To provide a baseline.
4. Position newborn in supine position, soft restraints; provide warmth under radiant warmer and have warm blankets available.	To provide maximum visualization and thermoregulation and to prevent chilling.
5. Clean abdomen by scrubbing.	To reduce number of bacteria present.
6. Attach monitor leads to infant.	To assess pulse and respiration.

*Exchange transfusion is a therapeutic procedure for hyperbilirubinemia of any etiology.

(continued)

Exchange Transfusion: Nursing Responsibilities *(continued)*

Nursing Action	Rationale
Objective: Prepare equipment.	
1. Have resuscitation equipment available (oxygen, bag and mask, intubation equipment, 10% glucose IV solution and sodium bicarbonate).	To provide life-support measures if necessary.
2. Obtain blood and check it with physician for type, Rh, and age.	To ensure using correct blood.
3. Attach blood tubing.	To allow infusion.
4. Apply blood warmer.	Blood temperature should be 37C prior to procedure to reduce chill.
5. Open exchange transfusion and umbilical vein trays. Pour prep solution into basins.	To maintain sterility.
6. Prepare gown and gloves for physician.	
Objective: Monitor infant status before and during procedure.	
Assess pulse, respirations, color, and activity state.	To recognize possible problems such as apnea, bradycardia, arrhythmia, or cardiac arrest and to provide data on neonate's response to treatment.

Objective: Record blood exchange and medications used.

1. Using blood exchange sheet, record time, amount of blood in, amount of blood out, medications and baby's response, and any other pertinent information.

Volume of donor blood given is 170 mL/kg of body weight. It replaces 85% of infant's own blood.

2. Inform physician when 100 mL of blood has been used.

Calcium gluconate is given IV after each 100 mL of blood if indicated to decrease cardiac irritability.

Objective: Assess newborn response after transfusion.

After the exchange, carefully monitor the following for 24–48 hr:

1. Vital signs

2. Neurologic signs (lethargy, increased irritability, jitteriness, convulsion)

3. Amount and color of urine (hematuria)

4. Presence of edema

5. Signs of necrotizing enterocolitis

6. Infection or hemorrhage at infusion site

7. Signs of increasing jaundice

8. Neurologic signs of kernicterus

To provide information on status of newborn and identify complications such as hypocalcemia, hyperkalemia, hypernatremia, hypoglycemia and acidosis, sepsis, shock, thrombus formation, and transfusion mismatch reaction.

(continued)

Exchange Tranfusion: Nursing Responsibilities *(continued)*

Nursing Action	Rationale
9. Calcium, glucose, and bilirubin levels	
10. Other complications such as hypokalemia, septicemia, shock, and thrombosis	
Objective: Prepare blood samples.	
Label tubes and send to laboratory with appropriate laboratory slips.	To follow routines of your institution.
Retype and cross-match 2 units of blood two hours post-exchange.	To provide for possible future exchange.
Objective: Record information on infant's record.	
Record infant's response during and after the exchange procedure.	Recording of infant's responses assists in identifying possible complications.

Fetal Heart Rate Auscultation

Nursing Action	Rationale
Objective: Assemble equipment.	
Obtain a fetoscope or Doppler.	Fetoscope is a special type of stethoscope that amplifies sound. Doppler uses ultrasound.
Objective: Prepare woman.	
Explain the procedure, indications for the procedure, and the information that will be obtained.	Explanation of the procedure decreases anxiety and increases relaxation.
Uncover the woman's abdomen.	
Objective: To use the fetoscope.	
Locate area of FHR using Leopold's maneuvers. Place the metal band of the fetoscope on your head; the diaphragm should extend out from your forehead.	The fetoscope is an older assessment tool; however, some clinicians prefer it because it is "natural" and does not rely on ultrasound. The metal band conducts sound.
Place the diaphragm on the woman's abdomen halfway between the umbilicus and symphysis pubis and in the midline.	The FHR is most likely to be heard in this area and over the fetal back. In LOA or ROA, the fetal back is located in this portion of the maternal abdomen. *(continued)*

Fetal Heart Rate Auscultation (*continued*)

Nursing Action	Rationale
Without touching the fetoscope listen carefully for the sounds of the fetal heart, which are called fetal heart tones (FHTs). If the FHTs are not heard, move the fetoscope laterally about an inch and then in a circle. Repeat in increasingly widening circles until the FHTs are heard.	
Objective: To use the Doppler.	
Place "ultrasonic gel" on the diaphragm of the Doppler.	Gel is used to maintain contact with the maternal abdomen and to enhance conduction of ultrasound.
Note: Some Dopplers have a plastic cap over the diaphragm that needs to be removed to expose the diaphragm.	
Place diaphragm on the woman's abdomen halfway between the umbilicus and symphysis pubis and in the midline.	The FHR is most likely to be heard in this area.
Listen carefully for the FHR. When using the Doppler, you may need to tilt the diaphragm slightly in order to hear the FHR. If tilting the diaphragm does not locate the FHR, move the Doppler in the same manner as described above.	Sound level may be controlled with a volume knob.
Objective: Differentiate maternal pulse from fetal	

heart rate.

For both methods:

Action	Rationale
Check the woman's pulse against the sounds heard. If the rates are the same, you have probably located maternal pulses (in abdominal vessels or in the placenta) and need to readjust the fetoscope or ultrasound device.	Ensures the FHR, not the woman's pulse, is being heard.
If the rates are not similar, count the FHR for 1 full minute. Note that the fetal heart has a double rhythm (like an adult's heart), and just one sound is counted. If the FHR is not found, move the fetoscope or ultrasound device laterally. Palpate for uterine contractions while you are auscultating FHR.	The FHR has the same "Lub dup" sound of adult heart sounds. The response of the FHR to uterine contractions is important in evaluating FHR changes.
Count FHR during a uterine contraction and continue for an additional 30 seconds to identify FHR response.	Counting during and just after the contraction evaluates fetal response to the contraction.
Determine FHR baseline by counting FHR for 30 to 60 seconds between uterine contractions to identify average baseline rate. Note if the rate is regular or irregular. If the rate changes (abruptly or gradually) recount for a brief period (5 or 10 seconds) to correctly identify an increasing or slowing rate.	The FHR baseline is the rate between contractions.
Tell parents what the FHR is; offer to help them listen if	Increases or decreases in the FHR need to be described as accurately as possible.

(continued)

Fetal Heart Rate Auscultation (continued)

Nursing Action	Rationale
they would like.	
Objective: Provide systematic evaluation.	
Auscultate between, during, and for 30 seconds following a uterine contraction. For low-risk women NAACOG (1990) recommends an auscultation frequency of every 1 hour in the latent phase, every 30 minutes in the active phase, and every 15 minutes in the second stage. For high-risk women the recommended frequency is every 30 minutes in the latent phase, every 15 minutes in the active phase, and every 5 minutes in the second stage.	Evaluation provides the opportunity to assess the fetal status and response to the labor process.
Objective: Record information on client's record.	
Document FHR data (rate and rhythm), characteristics of uterine activity and any actions taken as a result of the FHR.	Complete documentation is mandatory.

Sample nurse's entry:

0730 FHR 140 by auscultation, regular rhythm. Maternal pulse 78. UC q3min × 60 sec, strong. No increase or decrease in FHR noted during or following UC. J. Smith RN

Nurse's entry documents FHR rate, rhythm, and response to the labor process.

Sample nurse's entry for baseline and slowing of FHR after uterine contraction.

0730 FHR 136 by auscultation with slowing noted during the acme of UC and for 10 sec following the UC. Client turned to left side. Maternal pulse 80. FHR 140, regular rhythm with no decrease during or following the next two UC. UC q3min × 60 sec, strong. J. Smith RN

Nurse's entry documents FHR rate, response to UC, nursing intervention, and fetal response.

Fetal Monitoring: Electronic

Nursing Action	Rationale
Objective: Prepare woman.	
Explain the procedure, the indications for the EFM, and the information that will be obtained. Explain the monitor so that parents will know what they are seeing and hearing.	Explanation of the procedure decreases anxiety and increases relaxation.
Place the external fetal monitor. Turn on the monitor. Place two elastic belts around the woman's abdomen. Place the "toco" over the uterine fundus in the midline and secure it with a belt so that it fits snugly. Note the UC tracing. The resting tone tracing (without uterine contraction) should be recording on the 10 or 15 mm Hg pressure line.	The uterine fundus is the area of greatest contractility.
	If the tracing is on the 0 line, there may be a constant grinding noise.
Apply gel to the diaphragm of the ultrasound transducer. Place the diaphragm on the maternal abdomen between the umbilicus and symphysis pubis, in the midline. Listen for the FHR (which will have a "whip-like" sound). When FHR is located, attach the elastic belt snugly.	Ultrasonic gel is used to maintain contact with the maternal abdomen. The ultrasonic beam is directed toward the fetal heart.
	Firm contact is necessary to maintain a continuous tracing.

Objective: Identify the tracing.

Place the following information on the beginning of the fetal monitor paper: date, time, client name, gravida, para, membrane status, physician/CNM name. (Note: Each birthing area may have specific guidelines regarding additional information that is to be included.)

Assures accurate identification.

Objective: Evaluate EFM tracing.

For high-risk women, NAACOG (1988) recommends evaluating the EFM tracing every 15 minutes in the first stage, and every 5 minutes in the second stage. For low-risk women specific time intervals have not been recommended by NAACOG (now known as AWHONN). However, evaluation every 15–30 minutes in the first stage, and every 5–15 minutes in the second stage (as long as FHR has reassuring characteristics) is frequently done. The time interval for evaluation needs to be shortened if any nonreassuring characteristics occur.

Evaluation provides the opportunity to assess the fetal status and response to the labor process. Presence of reassuring characteristics is associated with good fetal outcome. Rapid identification of nonreassuring characteristics allows interventions to be initiated and then to determine the fetal response to the interventions.

Objective: Record information on client record.

Sample nurse's entry:
1/1/94 FHR BL 135–140. STV and LTV present. Two
0700   accelerations of 20 bpm × 20 sec with fetal

Nurse's entry documents reassuring FHR characteristics and response to UCs.

(continued)

Fetal Monitoring: Electronic (*continued*)

Nursing Action	Rationale
movement in 10 minutes. UC q 3 min × 50–60 sec of moderate intensity by palpation. No decelerations noted.	
Sample nurse's entry 0730 FHR BL 135–144. STV and LTV present. Late deceleration noted with decrease of FHR to 130 bpm for 20 sec. UC q 3 min × 50–60 sec of moderate intensity by palpation. Client turned to left side. No further deceleration with three subsequent UC. Two accelerations of 20 bpm × 20 sec noted with fetal movement. Client instructed to remain on left side.	Nurse's entry documents FHR rate, presence of variability, response of FHR to UC, the intervention used and subsequent positive fetal response to the intervention.

Fundal Assessment

Nursing Action	Rationale
Objective: Prepare woman.	
Explain procedure; have the woman void; position woman flat in bed with head comfortably positioned on a pillow; if the procedure is uncomfortable, woman may flex legs.	Having the woman void ensures that a full bladder is not causing any uterine atony. Having woman flat prevents falsely high assessment of fundal height. Flexing the legs relaxes the abdominal muscles. The uterus may be tender if frequent massage has been necessary.
Objective: Determine uterine firmness.	
Gently place one hand on the lower segment of the uterus; using the side of the other hand, palpate the abdomen until the top of the fundus is located. Determine whether the fundus is firm. If it is not firm, massage until firm.	Provides support for uterus. Provides a larger surface for palpation and is less uncomfortable for the woman. A firm fundus indicates that the muscles are contracted and bleeding will not occur.
Objective: Determine the height of the fundus.	
Measure the height of the top of the fundus in finger-breadths above, below, or at the umbilicus. (See accompanying figure.)	Fundal height gives information about the progress of involution.

(continued)

Fundal Assessment *(continued)*

Nursing Action	**Rationale**
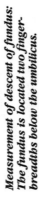	*Measurement of descent of fundus: The fundus is located two fingerbreadths below the umbilicus.*
Objective: Ascertain position.	
Determine whether fundus is deviated from the midline. If not in midline, locate position. Evaluate bladder for distention. Ascertain voiding pattern; use measuring device to measure urine output for next few hours (until normal elimination status is established).	Fundus may be deviated when bladder is full.
Objective: Correlate uterine status with lochia.	
Observe lochia for amount, presence of clots, color, and odor.	As normal involution occurs, the lochia decreases in amount and changes from rubra to serosa. Increased

amounts of lochia may be associated with uterine relaxation; failure to progress to next type of lochia may indicate uterine relaxation or infection.

Allows for consistency of reporting among care givers.

Objective: Record findings.

Fundal height is recorded in fingerbreadths; example: 2 FB ↓ U; 1 FB ↑ U.

If massage had been necessary it could be recorded as: Uterus: Boggy → firm c̄ light massage.

A complete note illustrating normal findings might be: Fundus firm, 1 FB ↓ U, lochia rubra, scant amount.

Gavage Feeding

Nursing Action

Objective: Prepare for smooth accomplishment of the procedure.

Gather necessary equipment including:

1. No. 5 or No. 8 Fr. feeding tube
2. 10–30 mL syringe
3. 1/4-in. paper tape
4. Stethoscope
5. Appropriate formula
6. Small cup of sterile water

Explain procedure to parents.

Rationale

Considerations in choosing size of catheter include size of the infant, area of insertion (oral or nasal), and rate of flow desired. The very small infant (less than 1600 g) requires a 5 Fr. feeding tube; an infant greater than 1600 g may tolerate a larger tube. Orogastric insertion is preferred over nasogastric insertion as most infants are obligatory nose breathers. If nasogastric insertion is used, a No. 5 catheter should be used to minimize airway obstruction. The size of the catheter will influence the rate of flow. The syringe is used to aspirate stomach contents prior to feeding, to inject air into the stomach for testing tube placement, and for holding measured amount of formula during feeding. Tape is used to mark tube for insertion depth as well as for securing tube during feeding. Stethoscope is needed to auscultate rush of air into stomach when testing tube placement.

Sterile water may be used to lubricate feeding tube when inserted nasally. With oral insertion, there are enough secretions in the mouth to lubricate the tube adequately. The cup of sterile water may also be used to test for placement by placing the end of the tube into the water to check for air bubbles from the lungs. However, this test may not be accurate as air may also be present in the stomach.

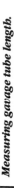

Measuring gavage tube length.

Objective: Insert tube accurately into stomach.

Position infant on back or side with head of bed elevated.

Take tube from package and measure the distance from the tip of the ear to the nose to the xiphoid process, and mark the point with a small piece of paper tape. (See accompanying figure.)

This position allows easy passage of the tube.

This measuring technique ensures enough tubing to enter stomach.

(continued)

Gavage Feeding (*continued*)

Nursing Action	Rationale
If inserting tube nasally, lubricate tip in cup of sterile water. Shake excess drops to prevent aspiration.	Water should be used, as opposed to an oil-based lubricant, in case the tube is inadvertently passed into a lung.
Stabilize infant's head with one hand, and pass the tube via the mouth (or nose) into the stomach, to the point previously marked. If the infant begins coughing or choking or becomes cyanotic or aphonic, remove the tube immediately.	Any signs of respiratory distress signal likelihood that tube has entered trachea. Orogastric insertion is less likely to result in passage into the trachea than nasogastric insertion.
If no respiratory distress is apparent, lightly tape tube in position, draw up 0.5–1.0 mL of air in syringe, and connect it to tubing. Place stethoscope over the epigastrium and briskly inject the air. (See accompanying figure.)	Nurse should hear a sudden rush of air as it enters stomach.

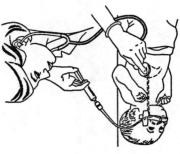

Auscultation for placement of gavage tube.

Aspirate stomach contents with syringe, and note amount, color, and consistency. Return residual to stomach unless otherwise ordered to discard it.	Residual formula should be evaluated as part of the assessment of infant's tolerance of gavage feedings. It is not discarded, unless particularly large in volume or mucoid in nature, because of the potential for causing an electrolyte imbalance.
If only a clear fluid or mucus is found upon aspiration and if any question exists as to whether the tube is in the stomach, the aspirate can be tested for pH.	Stomach aspirate tests in the 1–3 range for pH.
Objective: Introduce formula into stomach without complication.	
Hold infant for feeding or position on right side if infant cannot be held.	Positioning on side decreases the risk of aspiration in case of emesis during feeding.
Separate syringe from tube, remove plunger from barrel, reconnect barrel to tube, and pour formula into syringe.	Feeding should be allowed to flow in by gravity. It should not be pushed in under pressure with a syringe.
Elevate syringe 6–8 in. over infant's head. Allow formula to flow at slow, even rate.	Raising column of fluid increases force of gravity. Nurse may need to initiate flow of formula by inserting plunger of syringe into barrel just until formula is seen to enter feeding tube. Rate should be regulated to prevent sudden stomach distention, with possibility of vomiting and aspiration.

(continued)

Gavage Feeding (continued)

Nursing Action	Rationale
Continue adding formula to syringe until desired volume has been absorbed. Then rinse tubing with 2–3 mL sterile water.	Rinsing tube ensures that infant receives all of formula. It is especially important to rinse tube if it is going to be left in place, because this decreases risk of clogging and bacterial growth in tube.
Remove tube by loosening tape, folding the tube over on itself, and quickly withdrawing it in one smooth motion. If tube is to be left in, position it so that infant is unable to remove it.	Folding tube over on itself minimizes potential for aspiration of fluid, which would otherwise flow from tubing as it passes epiglottis. A tube left in place should be replaced at least every 24 hours.
Objective: Maximize feeding pleasure of infant.	
Whenever possible hold infant during gavage feeding. If it is too awkward to hold infant during feeding, be sure to take time for holding afterward.	Feeding time is important to infant's tactile sensory input.
Offer a pacifier to infant during feeding.	Infants fed for long periods by gavage can lose their sucking reflex. Sucking during feeding comforts and relaxes infant, making formula flow more easily. One study showed that infants allowed to suck during feedings were able to accept the nipple sooner and were discharged earlier than a control group of infants who did not suck during tube feedings.

Glucose Chemstrip Test Using Accu-Check II Machine

Nursing Action	Rationale
Objective: Assemble equipment.	
Gather the following equipment:	All necessary equipment must be ready to ensure that blood sample is collected at time and in manner necessary. Do not use needles because of danger of nicking periosteum. Warm heel for five to ten sec prior to heel stick with a warm wet wrap or specially designed chemical heat pad to facilitate flow of blood.
1. Lancet (do not use needles)	
2. Alcohol swabs	
3. 2 × 2 sterile gauze squares	
4. Small Band-Aid™	
5. Glucose strips and bottle	
6. Gloves	
Wash hands before and after touching infant and equipment; then apply gloves.	To implement universal precautions and prevent nosocomial infections.
Objective: Prepare infant's heel for procedure	
Select clear, previously unpunctured site. Clean site by rubbing vigorously with 70% isopropyl alcohol swab,	Selection of previously unpunctured site minimizes risk of infection and excessive scar formation. Friction produces

(continued)

Glucose Chemstrip Test Using Accu-Check II Machine (*continued*)

Nursing Action	Rationale
followed by dry gauze square. Grasp lower leg and heel so as to impede venous return slightly.	local heat, which aids vasodilation. Impeding venous return facilitates extraction of blood sample from puncture site.
Objective: Minimize trauma at puncture site.	
Blot dry site completely before lancing.	Alcohol is irritating to injured tissue and may also produce hemolysis.
With quick piercing motion, puncture lateral heel with microlancet, being careful not to puncture too deeply. (See accompanying figure.) Toes are acceptable sites if necessary.	The lateral heel is the site of choice because it precludes damaging the posterior tibial nerve and artery, plantar artery, and important longitudinally oriented fat pad of the heel, which in later years could impede walking. (See accompanying figure.) This is especially important for infant undergoing multiple heel stick procedures. Optimal penetration is 4 mm.
Objective: Ensure accurate blood sampling.	
After puncture is made, allow first drop of blood to touch both test pads on Chemstrip, making sure to cover both yellow and white squares completely. (See accompanying figure.)	Accuracy is greatest if the first drop of blood is used and only the squares are covered with blood.

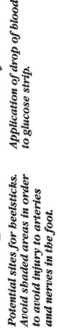

Application of drop of blood to glucose strip.

Wrong

Right

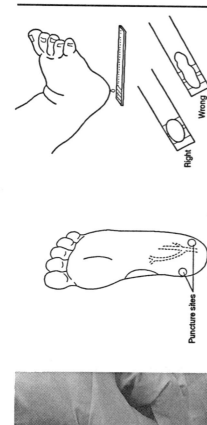

Potential sites for heelsticks. Avoid shaded areas in order to avoid injury to arteries and nerves in the foot.

Puncture sites

The first drop is usually discarded because it tends to be minutely diluted with tissue fluid from puncture.

(continued)

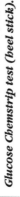

Glucose Chemstrip test (heel stick).

If Dextrostix reagent strip is used, first drop of blood is discarded.

Glucose Chemstrip Test Using Accu-Check II Machine *(continued)*

Nursing Action

Objective: Read reagent strip via Accu-Check II machine.

If using Accu-Check II machine,

Immediately press the TIME button. The meter will count to 60 but emit 3 high beeps on 57, 58, 59, then one low beep on 60. This is a warning to prepare for wiping the blood from the test strip. Wipe blood from test strips with clean dry cotton ball using moderate pressure when display reads 60. Do not leave any blood on test pad.

Machine will continue to count to 120 seconds. While meter is counting, turn test strip on side, with the test pads facing the On/Off button, and insert the reacted test strip into the test strip adapter. *The strip must be inserted before the display reads 120.*

When the display reads 120, a high beep will be emitted, followed by the blood sugar value on the display screen in mg/dL. Read the blood sugar value on the display screen.

Rationale

For accurate results, directions must be followed closely, and reagent strips must be fresh. False low readings may be caused by the following:

1. Inaccurate timing

2. Blood left on test strip

HHH = blood sugar > 500 mg/dL. Wait an additional minute and take the reacted test strip out of the meter and compare it to the color chart on the side of the Chemstrip bG vial to estimate results up to 800 mg/dL.

LLL = blood sugar is lower than the reading range of the instrument (less than 10 mg/dL). Values below 20 mg/dL have not been confirmed clinically.

Objective: Prevent excessive bleeding.

Apply folded gauze square to puncture site and secure firmly with bandage.

A pressure dressing should be applied to puncture site to stop bleeding.

Check puncture site frequently for first hour after sample.

Active infants sometimes kick or rub their dressings off and can bleed profusely from puncture site, especially if bandage becomes moist or is rubbed excessively against crib sheet.

Objective: Record infant's record.

Record test results. Report immediately any results under 45 mg/dL or over 175 mg/dL.

Recording of infant's results assists in identifying possible complications.

Heelstick for Newborns

Nursing Action	Rationale
Objective: Assemble and prepare equipment.	
Have following equipment available:	
2 × 2 or cotton balls Band-Aid™	
Micro lancet Gloves	
Alcohol and Betadine Heparinized capillary tubes (2)	
Heel warmer Lab slips and labels	
Objective: Prepare infant's heel for procedure.	
Wash hands.	Hand washing is the single most important step in the prevention of infection.
Apply heel warmer or moist, warm washcloth	Increases capillary dilatation and decreases venous stasis. Venous stasis results in higher hemoglobin and hematocrit values. Should be kept on heel 10–15 minutes.
Remove heel warmer	Decreases spread of infection.
Glove	Maintains universal precautions.
Cleanse foot with Betadine and allow to dry, then cleanse with alcohol.	Cleanses skin of bacteria.

Objective: Obtain blood for capillary hematocrit.

Use sterile microlancet stick. For proper puncture sites on lateral aspect of heel, see Procedure 10: Glucose Chemstrip Test.	Hematocrit is done to detect ratio of red blood cells (RBCs) to plasma in the blood. Use microlancet only one time. Be careful to avoid accidental puncture of medial plantar artery or injury to nerves.
Wipe away first drop of blood with a 2 × 2 or cotton ball.	First drop of blood is hemolyzed.
Obtain specimen as quickly as possible using a squeeze/ release technique.	Decreases trauma to surrounding tissues. Blood coagulates quickly.
Hold the heparinized capillary at a 45° angle to puncture site. Avoid air bubbles. Fill each tube two-thirds full and plug one end with clay. Put pressure on site with 2 × 2 until bleeding stops.	Air bubbles or clots may cause inaccurate results.
Apply Band-Aid if needed.	Protects from infection and further trauma.
Cuddle infant after procedure.	Provides sense of comfort and safety.
Send specimen to lab with slip, or run test on unit per agency policy.	

Objective: Report and record findings.

Record time, site of puncture, and infant's response.	Provides a permanent and continuous record of hematocrits drawn for lab quality assurance; decreases repeated punctures at one site and scar formation.

Installation of Ophthalmic Ilotycin Ointment

Nursing Action	Rationale
Objective: Provide newborn prophylactic eye care.	
Wash hands prior to instillation.	Prevents introduction of bacteria.
Clean infant's eyes of any drainage.	Removal of exudate allows instillation of ointment.
Retract lower eyelid outward with forefinger to allow instillation of 1/4-inch long strand of ointment along lower conjunctival surface, starting at inner canthus.	Maximizes absorption of ointment.
Repeat process on other eye.	
Instill only a single dose per eye.	Prophylaxis requires only a single dose.
Excess ointment may be wiped away after 1 minute (American Academy of Pediatrics 1992).	
Do not irrigate eyes.	Irrigation will remove ointment.
Assess for sensitivity reaction such as: edema, inflammation, drainage.	May interfere with ability to focus and the bonding process.

Inform parents about rationale for eye prophylaxis. Tell them that instillation can be done in the birthing area or admission nursery, that it may interfere with newborn's ability to focus on parents' faces, and that there may be temporary side effects.

Objective: Record completion of procedure.

Document the instillation of the prophylaxis eye medication

Preventive treatment of gonorrhea and *Chlamydia* infection, which can cause blindness. Required by law. Side effects usually disappear in 24 to 48 hours.

Provides a permanent record to meet the legal requirements.

Methods of Breast Pumping and Milk Storage

Breast Pumping—Manual Expression

Advantages

1. Collection container only equipment needed.
2. Technique easily learned.

Disadvantages

1. Time consuming.
2. Less effective than pumping.

Procedure

1. Assemble sterilized container and wash hands and breasts.
2. Perform gentle breast massage to stimulate the letdown reflex.
3. Position thumb and index finger about 1/2 inch behind nipple where milk sinuses are located.
4. Push fingers straight back toward chest and then squeeze them together with a slight rolling motion, lifting nipple outward. Avoid sliding fingers away from original position.
5. Rotate fingers around nipple to empty other milk sinuses. (Helpful hint: Practice technique on one breast while baby is nursing on other breast so infant will stimulate letdown reflex.)
6. Express milk into sterilized container.
7. Store as directed (see milk storage section).
8. Switch breasts as soon as flow in each breast decreases.

Breast Pumping—Using Breast Pumps

Advantages

1. Milk has a higher fat content when pumped with a breast pump than when expressed manually because more complete emptying of breasts allows access to hindmilk.

2. Increased volume obtained.

3. Less potential for milk contamination.

Disadvantages

1. More expensive—cost varies depending on equipment chosen.

2. Increased possibility of nipple trauma due to incorrect use or high pressures.

Procedures

Hand (Cylinder) Pump

1. Collect equipment. All equipment including hand pump, tubing, and collection bottles should be cleaned and/or sterilized between uses.

2. Wash hands and breasts.

3. Apply gentle massage or heat to breasts to stimulate flow of milk.

4. Alternate breasts as soon as flow decreases.

5. Place flange on breast and secure with one hand. If flange is not angled, mother should lean forward.

6. Suction is created by sliding outer cylinder away from breast, starting with short frequent pulls with other hand to initiate milk flow.

7. Empty breast milk into plastic storage container.

8. Repeat on opposite breast.

9. Store milk as directed.

(continued)

Methods of Breast Pumping and Milk Storage (*continued*)

Procedures

Battery-Operated Pumps

1. Follow steps 1 through 4 as for hand pump method.

2. Place flange on breast.

3. Turn on and regulate suction by depressing button or bar with one hand to achieve gentle, continuous suction.

4. Milk flows gently into storage container.

5. Repeat on other breast.

6. Store milk as directed.

7. Clean equipment.

Electric Pump

1. Follow steps 1 through 4 as for hand pump method.

2. After assembling pump, place flange over breast. If using double pump with Y connector, overall production is increased and pumping time is decreased by half.

3. Turn machine on with pressure setting on low and gradually increase pressure setting as tolerance permits.

4. Pump creates a rhythmic suck-release pattern closely approximating sucking action of baby.

5. Milk is expressed directly into storage container.

6. Seal and store milk as directed.

7. Clean equipment.

Milk Storage

1. Although milk may be stored in small plastic or glass bottles or disposable plastic bottle liners, the most recommended collection container is the rigid polypropylene plastic container, which maintains the stability of all constituents in human milk and is easier and safer to use.

2. Label milk with name, date, and time.

3. Once collected and sealed, milk may be stored in refrigerator for no more than 48 hours, freezer compartment of refrigerator for 2 weeks, or deep freezer for 6 months.

(continued)

Methods of Breast Pumping and Milk Storage (*continued*)

Milk Storage

4. Warm refrigerated milk in warm water for 10 to 15 minutes just prior to use. Do not microwave or heat on stove.

5. Discard all unused milk. Breast milk cannot be refrozen.

6. Freshly pumped milk can be added to already frozen milk by chilling it in refrigerator for 30 to 60 minutes prior to adding it to prevent the top layer of frozen breast milk from defrosting.

7. Thaw frozen milk in refrigerator up to 24 hours prior to use or in water just before feeding, gradually increasing temperature from cool to warm. Do not microwave or heat on stove.

8. Frozen breast milk may take on a yellow color which does not indicate spoilage.

9. If pumping and transporting milk, place milk in insulated pouch or cooler with ice to prevent spoilage.

RhIgG Administration

Nursing Action	Rationale
Objective: Confirm that Rh immune globulin (RhIgG) is indicated.	Sensitization occurs when an Rh negative woman is exposed to Rh positive blood. She develops antibodies to the Rh positive blood. These antibodies can attack the fetal red blood cells causing profound anemia. If both the direct and indirect Coombs' tests are negative, sensitization has not occurred and RhIgG is indicated.
Confirm that mother is Rh negative by checking her prenatal or intrapartal record. Then confirm that sensitization has not occurred—maternal indirect Coombs' negative.	
Confirm that infant is Rh positive. (A sample of the infant's cord blood is generally sent to the lab immediately after birth for typing and cross-matching.) If infant is Rh positive, confirm that sensitization has not occurred—direct Coombs' negative.	
Objective: Confirm that the woman does not have a history of allergy to immune globulin preparations.	
Review entries on medication allergies in client chart and ask woman specifically whether she has had any allergic reactions to medications, globulins, or blood products.	RhIgG is made from the plasma portion of blood. Allergic reactions are possible.

(continued)

RhIgG Administration (continued)

Nursing Action	Rationale
Objective: Explain purpose and procedure. Have consent signed.	
Many agencies require informed consent before administering RhIgG.	The woman should clearly understand the purpose of the procedure, its rationale, and the procedure itself, including any risks. Generally the primary side effects are erythema and tenderness at the injection site and allergic responses.
Objective: Obtain correct medication.	
RhIgG is available from the blood bank or pharmacy according to agency policy. Lot numbers for the drug and the cross match should be the same.	Because blood products are involved in the preparation careful verification is essential.
Objective: Confirm client identity and administer medication in deltoid muscle.	
Medication is administered intramuscularly within 72 hours of childbirth. The normal dose of 300 µg provides passive immunity following exposure of up to 15 mL of transfused RBCs or 30 mL of fetal blood. If a larger bleed is suspected (as in cases of severe abruptio	The medication causes passive immunity to occur and "tricks" the body into believing that it is not necessary to develop antibodies. Immunization is indicated any time there is a potential for maternal exposure to Rh positive blood. It is given prophylactically at 28 weeks' gestation,

placentae) additional doses may be administered at one time using multiple sites, or at regular intervals, as long as all doses are given within 72 hours of childbirth.

within 72 hours after the birth of an Rh positive Coombs' negative child, and following any spontaneous or therapeutic abortion, ectopic pregnancy, or amniocentesis.

Objective: Complete education for self-care.

Provide opportunities for the woman to ask questions and express concerns.

Many women, especially primigravidas, are not aware of the risks for an Rh positive fetus of a sensitized Rh negative mother. They must understand the importance of receiving medication for each pregnancy to ensure continued protection.

Objective: Complete client record.

Chart according to agency procedure. Most agencies chart lot number, route, dose, client education.

Provides a permanent record.

Sterile Vaginal Exam

Nursing Action	Rationale
Objective: Set the stage for the exam.	
Explain the procedure, indications for the exam, what the exam may feel like, that it may cause discomfort or pain, and information that may be obtained.	Explanation of exam can decrease the implied authority of the care giver, decrease anxiety, and increase relaxation.
Objective: Assemble and prepare equipment.	
Have following equipment easily accessible:	Examination is facilitated and can be done quickly.
• Sterile disposable gloves	
• Lubricant	
• Nitrazine test tape prior to first examination	
Objective: Position woman.	
Position woman with thighs flexed and abducted; instruct her to put heels of feet together.	Prevents contamination of area during examination and allows for visualization of external signs of labor progress.
Drape her so that only the perineum is exposed.	Provides as much privacy as possible.
Encourage woman to relax her muscles and legs during procedure.	

Objective: Use aseptic technique during examination.	
Inform woman prior to touching her. Use gentleness.	Communicates regard for the woman.
If leakage of fluid has been noted or if woman reports leakage of fluid, use Nitrazine test tape before doing vaginal exam.	Nitrazine test tape registers a change in pH if amniotic fluid is present (unless a lubricant has already been used).
Put on both gloves; using thumb and forefinger of nondominant hand, spread labia widely, insert well-lubricated second and index fingers of dominant hand into vagina until they touch the cervix.	Avoid contaminating hand by contact with anus; positioning of hand with wrist straight and elbow tilted downward allows fingertips to point toward umbilicus and find cervix.
If woman verbalizes discomfort, acknowledge it and apologize.	Maintain "realness" of the situation and decrease passive role of woman.
Objective: Determine status of fetal membranes.	
Palpate for movable bulging sac through the cervix; observe for expression of amniotic fluid during exam.	If intact, bag of waters feels like a bulge.
Objective: Determine status of labor progress during and after contractions.	
Carry out vaginal examination during and between contractions.	Examination varies. Assessment of dilatation is more accurate during contractions.

(continued)

Sterile Vaginal Exam (*continued*)

Nursing Action	Rationale
Objective: Identify degree of cervical dilatation.	
Palpate for opening or what appears as a depression in the cervix.	Estimation of the diameter of the depression identifies degree of dilatation.
Estimate diameter of cervical opening in centimeters (0–10 cm).	One finger represents approximately 1.5–2 cm cervical dilatation.
Objective: Identify degree of cervical effacement.	
Palpate the shortening of the surrounding circular ridge of tissue; estimate degree of shortening in percentages.	Effacement results from the lengthening of muscle fibers around the internal os as they are taken up into the lower uterine segment. The endocervix becomes part of the lower uterine segment.
Objective: Determine presentation and position of presenting part.	
As cervix opens, palpate for presenting part and identify its relationship to the maternal pelvis.	Presenting part is easier to palpate *through* a dilated cervix, and differentiation of landmarks is easier.
Objective: Determine station.	
Locate lowest portion of presenting part (excluding caput) (−5 to +5).	Identification of station provides information as to degree of descent.

Inform the woman that the exam is complete and remove your fingers.

Objective: Inform woman about progress in labor.

Discuss findings of the vaginal examination and correlate them to woman's progress in labor.

Assists in identifying progress and reinforces need for frequency of procedure.

Information is reassuring and supportive for woman and family.

Objective: Record information on client's record.

Record on labor record, eg, 4 cm 50% or 8 cm complete.

Nurse's entry documents progress of labor.

Suctioning of the Newborn

Nursing Action	Rationale
Objective: Assess infant.	If the infant shows signs of respiratory distress at birth the nurse must ensure patency of the airway.
Objective: Clear secretions from newborn's nose and/or oropharynx if respirations are depressed and/or if amniotic fluid was meconium stained.	
With DeLee mucus trap:	
Tighten the lid on the DeLee mucus trap or other suction device collection bottle.	Avoids spillage of secretions and prevents air from leaking out of lid.
Connect one end of DeLee tubing to low suction.	Provides suction.
Insert other end of tubing in newborn's nose or mouth 3 to 5 in.	Clears nasopharynx.
Continue suction as tube is removed.	Avoids redepositing secretions in newborn's nasopharynx.
Continue reinserting tube and providing suction for as long as fluid is aspirated.	Facilitates removal of secretions.
Note: Excessive suctioning can cause vagal stimulation, which causes decreased heart rate.	

Occasionally, the tube may be passed into the newborn's stomach to remove secretions or meconium that was swallowed before birth. If this is necessary, insert tube into newborn's mouth and then into stomach.	If meconium was present in amniotic fluid, the baby may have swallowed some.
	Secretions and/or meconium aspirate may be removed from newborn's stomach to decrease incidence of aspiration of stomach contents.
Provide suction and continue suction as tube is removed. Be careful not to aspirate the fluid yourself.	
With suction catheter:	
Using a #10 French catheter attached to suction, check negative pressure suction.	#10 French is correct size for oral suction of average-size newborn. Negative pressure not to exceed 80–100 cm H_2O.
Place catheter into newborn's mouth first. Place finger over control and gently rotate catheter as secretions are withdrawn with suction.	**No** suctioning episode should be longer than six seconds to prevent respiratory depression. Gentle rotation prevents trauma to mucous membranes.
Repeat suction of oropharynx if necessary to clear secretions.	Repeated suctioning must provide recovery time of at least 10–15 seconds to prevent respiratory depression.
Avoid deep suctioning, especially soon after birth.	Deep suction can stimulate the vagus nerve, causing a decrease in heart rate.
With bulb syringe:	
If using bulb syringe, deflate the bulb prior to inserting it into the mouth and/or the nose.	This prevents blowing the contents further into the nose and/or throat.

(continued)

Suctioning of the Newborn (continued)

Nursing Action	Rationale
Immediately after birth, insert bulb into mouth first and then into the nares.	Suctioning after birth requires clearing the mouth first to prevent aspiration of contents. Then suction the nares of birth secretions.
For routine suctioning, insert bulb into the nares, then corners of the mouth.	Infants can show signs of respiratory distress if the nose is congested, since infants are obligatory nose breathers. Don't force bulb into the nares and/or mouth.
Gently release the compressed bulb.	Provides suction that will draw the secretions into bulb.
Empty the bulb of secretions by squeezing it hard onto a cloth or paper towel.	
Reassess the infant's respiratory status.	It may take several times before nares and/or mouth are cleared. Take care not to traumatize the infant. If color change or bradycardia occur, oxygen or resuscitative procedures may be needed.
Clean the inside and outside of the bulb after using it by rinsing with clear water.	Dry secretions become a medium for bacterial growth.
Objective: Record information on client's record.	
Record procedure, method, and how infant tolerated it.	
Document amount, color, consistency of aspirate, and whether specimen was sent to lab for analysis.	Provides documentation of intervention and status at birth.

Temperature Stabilization of the Newborn

Nursing Action	Rationale
Objective: Prepare warming equipment.	
Prewarm incubator or radiant warmer. Have warmed towels/lightweight blankets available	
Maintain birthing room at 22C (71F) with relative humidity of 60% to 65%.	Change from warm, moist intrauterine environment to cool, dry, drafty environment stresses the immature thermoregulation mechanisms of newborn.
Objective: Establish a stable temperature after birth.	
Wipe newborn free of blood and excessive vermix, especially from the head, with prewarmed towels.	Prevents loss of body heat from large surface area through evaporation.
Place newborn under radiant warmer.	Creates a heat-gaining environment.
Wrap newborn in prewarmed blanket and transfer to mother.	Reduces convective heat loss. Facilitates immediate maternal-infant contact without compromising infant thermoregulation.
Place skin-to-skin with mother under warmed blanket.	Skin-to-skin contact with mother or father acts to maintain newborn's temperature.

(continued)

Temperature Stabilization of the Newborn (*continued*)

Nursing Action	Rationale
Objective: Maintain stable infant temperature.	
Diaper newborn and place hat on head. Place newborn uncovered (except for diaper and hat) under radiant warmer.	Radiant heat warms outer surface skin so skin needs to be exposed.
Tape servocontrol probe on infant's anterior abdominal wall (metal side next to skin) and cover with aluminum heat deflector patch.	Aluminum cover prevents heating of probe directly and overheating of infant. Turn heater to servocontrol mode with abdominal skin temperature maintained at 36.5C–37C.
Monitor infant's axillary and skin probe temperature per institution protocol.	Rechecking temperature ensures that it is within desired range. Temperature indicator on the radiant warmer continually displays baby's probe temperature so that nurse can check baby's axillary temperature to ensure that the machine accurately reports baby's temperature.
Once infant's temperature reaches 37C (98.6F), remove infant from radiant warmer. Dress infant in T-shirt, diaper, and stocking hat then wrap in two blankets (called double wrap). Place in open crib. Recheck axillary temperature in one hour.	It is important to monitor infant's ability to maintain own thermoregulation.

Objective: Rewarm infant gradually if temperature < 36.1C (97F)	
Assess temperature frequently. Check axillary temperature per birthing center routine usually every 2 to 4 hours.	Early detection of hypothermia, which predisposes infant to cold stress.
Place unclothed infant with diaper under radiant warmer with servocontrol probe on abdomen.	Rapid heating leads to hyperthermia.
Gradually rewarm infant back to normal temperature.	Hyperthermia caused by too-rapid warming is associated with apnea, increased insensible water loss, and increased metabolic rate.
Recheck temperature in 30 minutes, then hourly.	
Once infant's temperature reaches 37C (98.6F), remove from heater, dress, double-wrap with hat on, and place in open crib. Recheck temperature in 1 hour.	
Objective: Prevent drops in baby's temperature.	
Keep infant clothing and bedding dry.	
Double-wrap with hat on.	Prevents loss of heat by conduction, convection, radiation, and evaporation.
Use radiant warmer during procedures.	
Reduce exposure to drafts.	
Warm objects coming in contact with infant, eg, stethoscopes.	
Encourage mother to snuggle with infant under blankets or breastfeed with light cover over infant.	

REFERENCES

American Academy of Pediatrics: *Guidelines for Perinatal Care,* 3d ed. Chicago: American Academy of Pediatrics, 1992.

Luegenbiehl DL, Brophy GH, Artique GS, et al: Standardized assessment of blood loss. *Matern Child Nurs* July/August 1990; 15:241.

NAACOG OGN Nursing Practice Resource: Fetal heart rate auscultation. March 1990.

NAACOG Statement. Nursing Responsibilities in implementing intrapartum fetal heart rate monitoring. October 1988.

Common Abbreviations in Maternal-Newborn Nursing

Accel	Acceleration of fetal heart rate
AC	Abdominal circumference
AFAFP	Amniotic fluid alpha fetoprotein
AFP	α-fetoprotein
AFV	Amniotic fluid volume
AGA	Average for gestational age
AID or AIH	Artificial insemination donor (H designates mate is donor)
ARBOW	Artificial rupture of bag of waters
AROM	Artificial rupture of membranes
BAT	Brown adipose tissue (brown fat)
BL	Baseline (fetal heart rate baseline)
BOW	Bag of waters
BPD	Biparietal diameter *or* Bronchopulmonary dysplasia
BPM	Beats per minute
BPP	Biophysical profile
BSE	Breast self-examination
BSST	Breast self-stimulation test
CC	Chest circumference *or* Cord compression
C–H	Crown-to-heel length
CID	Cytomegalic inclusion disease
CMV	Cytomegalovirus
CNM	Certified nurse-midwife
CPD	Cephalopelvic disproportion
CRL	Crown-rump length
C/S	Cesarean section or (C-section)
CST	Contraction stress test
CVS	Chorionic villus sampling
decels	deceleration of fetal heart rate
DIC	Disseminated intravascular coagulation
dil	dilatation
DTR	Deep tendon reflexes
ECHMO	Extracorporeal membrane oxygenator
EDB	Estimated date of birth
EDC	Estimated date of confinement
EFM	Electronic fetal monitoring
ELF	Elective low forceps

epis	Episiotomy
FAD	Fetal activity diary
FAS	Fetal alcohol syndrome
FB	Fingerbreadth
FBM	Fetal breathing movements
FBS	Fetal blood sample *or* fasting blood sugar test
FECG	Fetal electrocardiogram
FHR	Fetal heart rate
FHT	Fetal heart tones
FL	Femur length
FM	Fetal movement
FMD	Fetal movement diary
FSH	Follicle-stimulating hormone
G or grav	Gravida
GDM	Gestational diabetes mellitus
GTPAL	Gravida, term, preterm, abortion, living children
HA	Head-abdominal rates
HAI	Hemagglutination-inhibition test
HC	Head compression
hCG	Human chorionic gonadotrophin
hCS	Human chorionic somatomammotrophin (same as hPL)
HMD	Hyaline membrane disease
hPL	Human placental lactogen
HVH	Herpes virus hominis
IDDM	Insulin-dependent diabetes mellitus
IDM	Infant of a diabetic mother
IUD	Intrauterine device
IUFD	Intrauterine fetal death
IUGR	Intrauterine growth retardation
LADA	Left-acromion-dorsal-anterior
LADP	Left-acromion-dorsal-posterior
LBW	Low birth weight
LDR	Labor, delivery, and recovery room
LGA	Large for gestational age
LH	Luteinizing hormone
LMA	Left-mentum-anterior
LML	Left mediolateral (episiotomy)
LMP	Last menstrual period *or* Left-mentum-posterior
LMT	Left-mentum-transverse

LOA	Left-occiput-anterior
LOF	Low outlet forceps
LOP	Left-occiput-posterior
LOT	Left-occiput-transverse
L/S	Lecithin/sphingomyelin ratio
LSA	Left-sacrum-anterior
LSP	Left-sacrum-posterior
LST	Left-sacrum-transverse
LTV	Long-term variability
MAS	Meconium aspiration syndrome
mec	Meconium
mec st	Meconium stain
ML	Midline (episiotomy)
MSAFP	Maternal serum alpha fetoprotein
multip	Multipara
NEC	Necrotizing enterocolitis
NIDDM	Noninsulin-dependent diabetes mellitus
NSCST	Nipple stimulation contraction stress test
NST	Nonstress test *or* nonshivering thermogenesis
NSVD	Normal sterile vaginal delivery
NTD	Neural tube defects
NTZ	Neutral thermal zone
OA	Occiput anterior
OF	Occipitofrontal diameter of fetal head
OFC	Occipitofrontal circumference
OM	Occipitomental (diameter)
OP	Occiput posterior
P	Para
Pap smear	Papanicolaou smear
PDA	Patent ductus arteriosus
PEEP	Positive end-expiratory pressure
PG	Phosphatidyglycerol *or* Prostaglandin
PI	Phosphatidylinositol
PIH	Pregnancy-induced hypertension
Pit	Pitocin
PKU	Phenylketonuria
PPHN	Persistent pulmonary hypertension
Preemie	Premature infant
Primip	Primapara
PROM	Premature rupture of membranes
PUBS	Percutaneous umbilical blood sampling
RADA	Right-acromion-dorsal-anterior

RADP	Right-acromion-dorsal-posterior
RDS	Respiratory distress syndrome
RIA	Radioimmune assay
RLF	Retrolental fibroplasia
RMA	Right-mentum-anterior
RMP	Right-mentum-posterior
RMT	Right-mentum-transverse
ROA	Right-occiput-anterior
ROM	Rupture of membranes
ROP	Right-occiput-posterior, *or* retinopathy of prematurity
ROT	Right-occiput-transverse
RSA	Right-sacrum-anterior
RSP	Right-sacrum-posterior
RST	Right-sacrum-transverse
SFD	Small for dates
SGA	Small for gestational age
SIDS	Sudden infant death syndrome
SMB	Submentobregmatic diameter
SOB	Suboccipitobregmatic diameter
SRBOW	Spontaneous rupture of the bag of waters
SROM	Spontaneous rupture of the membranes
STD	Sexually transmitted disease
STS	Serologic test for syphilis, Sexually transmitted serology
STV	Short-term variability
SVE	Sterile vaginal exam
TC	Thoracic circumference
TCM	Transcutaneous monitoring
TORCH	Toxoplasmosis, rubella, cytomegalovirus, herpesvirus hominis type 2
ū	umbilicus
UA	Uterine activity
UAC	Umbilical artery catheter
UAU	Uterine activity units
UC	Uterine contraction
UPI	Uteroplacental insufficiency
U/S	Ultrasound
VBAC	Vaginal birth after cesarean
VDRL	Venereal Disease Research Laboratories
WIC	Supplemental food program for Women, Infants, and Children

Conversion of Pounds and Ounces to Grams

	OUNCES 0	1	2	3	4	5	6	7	8	9	10	11	12	13	14	OUNCES 15
0	—	28	57	85	113	142	170	198	227	255	283	312	340	369	397	425
1	454	482	510	539	567	595	624	652	680	709	737	765	794	822	850	879
2	907	936	964	992	1021	1049	1077	1106	1134	1162	1191	1219	1247	1276	1304	1332
3	1361	1389	1417	1446	1474	1503	1531	1559	1588	1616	1644	1673	1701	1729	1758	1786
4	1814	1843	1871	1899	1928	1956	1984	2013	2041	2070	2098	2126	2155	2183	2211	2240
5	2268	2296	2325	2353	2381	2410	2438	2466	2495	2523	2551	2580	2608	2637	2665	2693
6	2722	2750	2778	2807	2835	2863	2892	2920	2948	2977	3005	3033	3062	3090	3118	3147
7	3175	3203	3232	3260	3289	3317	3345	3374	3402	3430	3459	3487	3515	3544	3572	3600
8	3629	3657	3685	3714	3742	3770	3799	3827	3856	3884	3912	3941	3969	3997	4026	4054
9	4082	4111	4139	4167	4196	4224	4252	4281	4309	4337	4366	4394	4423	4451	4479	4508
P 10	4536	4564	4593	4621	4649	4678	4706	4734	4763	4791	4819	4848	4876	4904	4933	4961
O 11	4990	5018	5046	5075	5103	5131	5160	5188	5216	5245	5273	5301	5330	5358	5386	5415
U 12	5443	5471	5500	5528	5557	5585	5613	5642	5670	5698	5727	5755	5783	5812	5840	5868
N 13	5897	5925	5953	5982	6010	6038	6067	6095	6123	6152	6180	6209	6237	6265	6294	6322
D 14	6350	6379	6407	6435	6464	6492	6520	6549	6577	6605	6634	6662	6690	6719	6747	6776
S 15	6804	6832	6860	6889	6917	6945	6973	7002	7030	7059	7087	7115	7144	7172	7201	7228
16	7257	7286	7313	7342	7371	7399	7427	7456	7484	7512	7541	7569	7597	7626	7654	7682
17	7711	7739	7768	7796	7824	7853	7881	7909	7938	7966	7994	8023	8051	8079	8108	8136
18	8165	8192	8221	8249	8278	8306	8335	8363	8391	8420	8448	8476	8504	8533	8561	8590
19	8618	8646	8675	8703	8731	8760	8788	8816	8845	8873	8902	8930	8958	8987	9015	9043
20	9072	9100	9128	9157	9185	9213	9242	9270	9298	9327	9355	9383	9412	9440	9469	9497
21	9525	9554	9582	9610	9639	9667	9695	9724	9752	9780	9809	9837	9865	9894	9922	9950
22	9979	10007	10036	10064	10092	10120	10149	10177	10206	10234	10262	10291	10319	10347	10376	10404

Cervical Dilatation Assessment Aid

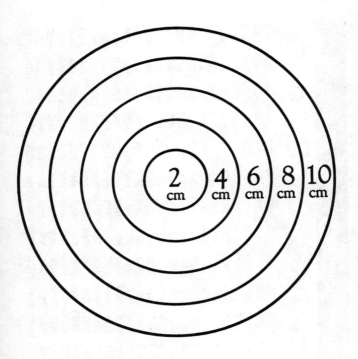

*Actions and Effects of Selected Drugs During Breastfeeding**

Anticholinergics

Atropine: May cause hyperthermia in the newborn; may decrease maternal milk supply

Anticoagulants

Coumarin derivatives (warfarin, Coumadin): Only small amount in breast milk; check PTT
Heparin: Relatively safe to use; check PTT
Phenindione (Hedulin): Passes easily into breast milk; neonate may have increased prothrombin time and PTT

Anticonvulsants

Phenytoin (Dilantin), phenobarbital: Generally considered safe; if high doses of phenobarbital are ingested, may cause drowsiness; short-acting phenobarbiturates (secobarbital) preferred, as they appear in lower concentration in milk

Antihistamines

Diphenhydramine (Benadryl), phenira-mine (Dimetane), Coricidin, Drexoral: May cause decreased milk supply; infant may become drowsy, irritable, or have tachycardia

Antimetabolites

Unknown, probably long-term anti-DNA effect on the infant; potentially very toxic

Antimicrobials

Ampicillin: Skin rash, candidiasis, diarrhea
Chloramphenicol: Possible bone marrow depression; gray syndrome; refusal of breast
Methacycline: Possible inhibition of bone growth; may cause discoloration of the teeth; use should be avoided
Sulfonamides: May cause hyperbilirubinemia; use contraindicated until infant over 1 month old
Penicillin: Possible allergic response; candidiasis
Metronidazole (Flagyl): Posssible neurologic disorders or blood dyscrasias; delay

*Based on data from Kacew S: Adverse effects of drugs and chemicals in breast milk on the nursing infant. *J Clin Pharmacol* 1993;33:213–331: Riordan J. Auerbach KG: *Breastfeeding and Human Lactation.* Boston: Jones and Bartlett, 1993, pp 135–166.

breastfeeding for 12 hours after dose

Aminoglycosides: May cause ototoxicity or nephrotoxicity if given for more than two weeks

Tetracycline: Long-term use and large doses should be avoided; may cause tooth staining or inhibition of bone growth

Quinolones (synthetic antibiotics): Can cause arthropathies

Antithyroids

Thiouracil: Contraindicated during lactation; may cause goiter or agranulocytosis

Barbiturates

May produce sedation

Phenothiazines: May produce sedation

Bronchodilators

Aminophylline: May cause insomnia or irritability in the infant

Ephedrine, cromolyn (Intal): Relatively safe

Caffeine

Excessive consumption may cause jitteriness

Cardiovascular

Propranolol (Inderal): May cause hypoglycemia; possibility of other blocking effects, especially if infant has renal or liver dysfunction

Quinidine: May cause arrhythmias in infant

Reserpine (Serpasil): Nasal stuffiness, lethargy, or diarrhea in infant

Methyldopa: Increase in milk volume

Corticosteroids

Adrenal suppression may occur with long-term administration of doses greater than 10 mg/day.

Diuretics

Furosemide (Lasix): Not excreted in breast milk

Thiazide diuretics (Esidrix, HydroDIURIL, Oretic): Safe but can cause dehydration, reduce milk production

Heavy metals

Gold: Potentially toxic

Mercury: Excreted in the milk and hazardous to infant

Hormones

Androgens: Suppress lactation

Thyroid hormones: May mask hypothyroidism

Laxatives

Cascara: May cause diarrhea in infant

Milk of magnesia: Relatively safe

Phenolphthalein: May cause diarrhea in infant

Narcotic analgesics

Codeine: Accumulation may lead to neonatal depression

Meperidine: May lead to neonatal depression

Morphine: Long-term use may cause newborn addiction

Nonnarcotic analgesics, NSAIDs

Salicylates (aspirin): Safe after first week of life; monitor protein

Acetaminophen (Tylenol): Relatively safe for short-term analgesia

Propoxyphene (Darvon): May cause sleepiness and poor nursing in infant

Ibuprofen (Motrin): Safe

Oral Contraceptives:

Combined estrogen/progestin pills: Significantly decrease milk supply; may alter milk composition; may cause gynecomastia in male infants

Progestin only: Safe if started after lactation is established

Radioactive materials for testing

Gallium citrate (^{67}G): Insignificant amount excreted in breast milk; no nursing for 2 weeks

Iodine: Contraindicated; may affect infant's thyroid gland

^{125}I: Discontinue nursing for 48 hours

^{131}I: Nursing should be discontinued until excretion is no longer significant; after a test dose, nursing may be resumed after 24 to 36 hours; after a treatment dose, nursing may be resumed after 2 to 3 weeks

$^{99}Technetium$-99m: Discontinue nursing for 3 days (half-life = 6 hours)

Sedatives/Tranquilizers

Diazepam (Valium): May accumulate to high levels; may increase neonatal jaundice; may cause lethargy

Lithium carbonate: Controversial; may cause neonatal flaccidity and hypotonia

Substance abuse

Alcohol: Potential motor developmental delay; mild sedative effect

Amphetamines: Controversial; may cause irritability, poor sleeping

Cocaine, crack: Extreme irritability, tachycardia, vomiting, apnea

Marijuana: Drowsiness

Selected Maternal–Newborn Laboratory Values

Normal Maternal Laboratory Values

Test	Non-pregnant Values	Pregnant Values
Hematocrit	37%–47%	32%–42%
Hemoglobin	12–16 gm/dL*	10–14 gm/dL*
Platelets	150,000–350,000/mm³	Significant increase three to five days after birth (predisposes to thrombosis)
Partial thrombo-plastin time (PTT)	12–14 seconds	Slight decrease in pregnancy and again in labor (placental site clotting)
Fibrinogen	250 mg/dL	400 mg/dL
Serum glucose: Fasting 2-hour post-prandial	 70–80 mg/dL 60–110 mg/dL	 65 mg/dL Less than 140 mg/dL
Total protein	6.7–8.3 gm/dL	5.5–7.5 gm/dL
White blood cell total	4500–10,000/mm³	5000–15,000/mm³
Polymorpho-nuclear cells	54%–62%	60%–85%
Lymphocytes	38%–46%	15%–40%

*at sea level

Normal Neonatal Laboratory Values

Test	Normal Values
Hematocrit	51% to 56%
Hemoglobin	16.5 gm/dL (cord blood)
Platelets	150,000–400,000/mm^3
White blood cell total	18,000/mm^3
White blood cell differential:	
Bands	1600/mm^3 (9%)
Polymorphonuclear (segs)	9400/mm^3 (52%)
Eosinophils	400/mm^3 (2.2%)
Basophils	100/mm^3 (0.6%)
Lymphocytes	5500/mm^3 (31%)
Monocytes	1050/mm^3 (5.8%)
Serum glucose	40–80 mg/dL
Serum electrolytes:	
Sodium	135–147 mEq/L
Potassium	4–6 mEq/L
Chloride	90–114 mEq/L
Carbon dioxide	15–25 mEq/L
Bicarbonate	18–23 mEq/L
Calcium	7–10 mg/dL

*at sea level

Spanish Translations of English Phrases[1]

This Appendix includes phrases you might find helpful in working with families during pregnancy, labor and birth, and after the birth. There are many ways to phrase questions. We have chosen some statements we consider essential and have tried to phrase them in a straightforward way. The phrases are designed to help you in situations in which translation is not possible at the moment.

This list begins with introductory statements, which are presented in a logical conversational flow. The remaining phrases are arranged according to the phases of pregnancy and birth during which they are most applicable.

Essential Introductory Phrases	**Frases Introductoras Esenciales**
Hello.	Hola.
I am a nurse.	Soy enfermera (enfermero).[2]
I am a student nurse.	Soy estudiante de enfermería.
My name is _____	Mi nombre es _____ Me llamo _____
What is your name?	¿Cuál es su nombre? ¿Cómo se llama?
What name should I call you?	¿Cómo quiere que la llamemos? ¿Cómo quiere ser llamada?
Thank you.	Gracias.
Please.	Por favor.
Is someone here with you?	¿Hay alquien aquí con usted?
Does he (she) speak English?	¿Habla él (ella) English?
Goodbye.	Adiós

1. Prepared by Elizabeth Medina, PhD, Associate Professor of Spanish, Regis University, Denver, Colorado
2. In Spanish, nouns that end in *a* indicate female gender. Nouns that end in *o* indicate male gender.

Phrases for the Antepartal Period

Frases para el Periodo Prenatal

Are you taking any medications now?

¿Está tomando algunas medicinas ahora?

Show me the medicine bottles please.

Por favor, muéstreme los frascos.

Have you ever had trouble with your blood pressure?

¿Ha tenido problemas alguna vez con la presión arterial?

When was the first day of your last period?

¿Cuál fue el primer día de su última regla?
¿Cuál fue el primer día de su última menstruación?

Have you had any spotting or bleeding since your last period?

¿Ha sangrado o ha tenido manchas de sangre desde su última regla?

Have you been on birth control pills?

¿Ha estado tomando píldoras anticonceptivas?

When did you stop taking them?

¿Cuándo dejó de tomarlas?

Do you have an intrauterine device (IUD)?

¿Usa un aparato intrauterino?

How many times have you been pregnant?

¿Cuántas veces ha estado usted embarazada?

Are you having any problems with your pregnancy?

¿Tiene problemas con su embarazo?

Is there anything that is worrying you?

¿Hay algo o alguna cosa que la preocupe?

I would like to take your blood pressure.

Quisiera tomarle la presión arterial.

I would like to take your pulse.

Quisiera tomarle el pulso.

I would like to take your temperature.

Quisiera tomarle la temperatura.

I would like to listen to your heart and lungs.

Quisiera escucharle el corazon y los pulmones.

I would like to check your uterus.

Quisiera examinarle el útero.

Would you please urinate in this cup and leave it in the bathroom.

Puede orinar en este vaso y dejarlo en el baño.

Phrases for the Antepartal Period

Please stand up.

Please sit down.

Please lie down.

Frases para el Periodo Prenatal

Por favor, levántese.

Por favor, siéntese.

Por favor, acuéstese.

Phrases Related to Client Safety

I would like to talk to you alone.

Are you safe at home?

Are you afraid of your partner?

During your pregnancy has your partner hit, slapped, kicked, or punched you?

How many times?

Do you have someone for support?

Frases Relacionadas con la Seguridad del Cliente

Quisiera hablar a solas con usted.

¿Sufre de peligros en casa?

¿Le tiene miedo a su compañero?

Durante su embarazo, ¿la ha golpeado? ¿la ha abofeteado? ¿la ha pateado? o ¿le ha dado puñetazos?

¿Cuántas veces?

¿Cuénta con alguien que la pueda ayudar?

Questions the Mother or Father May Ask

How big is my baby?

How much does the baby weigh now?

When will I feel my baby move?

Posibles Preguntas que Madres y Padres Hacen

¿De qué tamaño es el (la) bebé ahora?

¿Cuánto pesa el bebé ahora?

¿Cuándo lo (la) voy a sentir moverse?

Phrases for the Intrapartal Period

Note: Review the Essential Introductory Phrases for beginning conversation.

Are you having labor pains?

Are you having contractions?

Are you having pain?

Frases Durante el Parto

Nota: Repase las frases introductoras para comenzar una conversación.

¿Tiene dolores de parto?

¿Tiene contracciones?

¿Tiene dolores?

Phrases for the Intrapartal Period

Frases Durante el Parto

Do you need medicine for pain?

¿Necesita medicina para el dolor?

Do you need to urinate?

¿Necesita orinar?

This is a bedpan to urinate in.

Aquí tiene el bacín (la chata) (el pato) para orinar.

Can I help you to the bathroom?

¿La ayudo a ir al baño?

Do you need to have a bowel movement?

¿Necesita mover el vientre (obrar)? Necesita "hacer caca"—coloquial

Has your bag of water broken?

¿Se le ha roto la bolsa de aqua(s)?

Have you had any bright red bleeding during your pregnancy?

¿Ha tenido algún sangramiento de color rojo durante su embarazo?

How many births have you had?

¿Cuántos niños le han nacido?

I need to do a vaginal examination.

Necesito hacerle un examen vaginal.

I will help you.

La voy a ayudar.

I will stay with you.

Me quedaré con usted.

Please pant. I will show you how.

Por favor, jadee. Le voy a mostrar cómo.

Please do not push.

No puje ahora.

Push now.

Puje ahora.

Stop pushing.

Pare de pujar.
No puje más.

The doctor needs to do a cesarean birth.

El doctor le va a hacer una operación cesárea.

This is medicine for your pain. You will feel better soon.

Esta medicina es para el dolor. Va a sentirse mejor pronto.

When is your baby supposed to be born?

¿Cuándo está supuesto a nacer el bebé?

January	February	enero	febrero
March	April	marzo	abril
May	June	mayo	junio
July	August	julio	agosto
September	October	septiembre	octubre
November	December	noviembre	diciembre

Phrases for the Intrapartal Period

Frases Durante el Parto

What is your doctor's name?

¿Cuál es el nombre de su doctor?

What is your midwife's name?

¿Cuál es el nombre de su comadrona (partera)?

Your baby is having a little trouble now.

El bebé está pasando por algunos problemas.
El bebé está sufriendo algunas dificultades.

I need to put this oxygen mask on you. It will help your baby. It may smell funny, but it is ok.

Le voy a poner esta máscara de oxígeno. Va a ayudar al bebé. Huele extraño, pero no hay problemas.

Please turn on your left side.

Por favor voltéese al lado izquierdo.

Please turn on your right side.

Por favor voltéese al lado derecho.

Your baby is ok.

El bebé está bien.

Phrases for the Postpartal Period and the Newborn Area

Frases para el Periodo Despues del Parto y el Area del Recien Nacido

Note: Review the Essential Introductory Phrases for beginning conversation.

Nota: Repase las frases introductoras para comenzar una conversación.

Are you hungry?

¿Tiene hambre?

Are you thirsty?

¿Tiene sed?

Are you cold?

¿Tiene frío?

Are you tired?

¿Está cansada?

I am going to put antibiotic ointment in the baby's eyes. It will help protect your baby from some infections.

Le voy a poner al bebé un ungüento antibiótico alrededor de los ojos.
Lo (la) va a proteger contra infecciones.

I am going to take some blood from your baby's foot to check the blood sugar and hemocrit.

Le voy a sacar sangre del pie al bebé para determinar el azúcar de la sangre y el hematocrítico.

If your baby begins to spit up, please turn him (her) on his (her) side.

Si el bebé comienza a vomitar, colóquelo (colóquela) de costado.

**Phrases for the
Postpartal Period and
the Newborn Area**

**Frases para el Periodo
Despues del Parto y
el Area del Recien Nacido**

It may help to position your
baby like this.

Lo (la) ayudará—si lo
coloca así.
Lo (la) ayudaría—si lo
colocara así.

I would like to suggest that
you clean your nipples
this way before you
breastfeed your baby.

Es bueno que se lave los
pezones de esta manera
antes de darle el pecho
al bebé.

I would like to suggest that
you clean your baby's
cord this way.

Es mejor para el bebé que
le lave el ombligo de esta
manera.

I would like to suggest that
you bathe your baby this
way.

Es mejor que lo (la) bañe de
esta manera.

I would like to suggest that
you clean your baby's
penis this way.

Es mejor que le limpie el
pene así.

I would like you to fold the
diaper this way.

Le sugiero que doble el
pañal así.

I would like to suggest that
you fasten the diaper this
way.

Le sugiero que asegure el
pañal así.

I would like to suggest that
you take the baby's tem-
perature this way.

Tómele la temperatura así.

I need to check your breasts,
your uterus, your flow,
your stitches, your legs
and feet.

Necesito examinarle los
pechos, el útero, el flujo,
los puntos, las piernas y
los pies.

I need to feel your uterus.

Necesito examinarle el útero.

I need to massage your
uterus.

Necesito darle un masaje en
la región del útero.

Place your baby on its side.

Coloque al bebé de costado.

Place the baby's used
diaper here.

Coloque aquí los pañales
usados.

Please rub your uterus every
half hour to keep it firm.
I will show you how.

Necesita darse un masaje en
la región del útero cada
media hora para manten-
erlo firme. Le voy a
mostrar cómo.

Phrases for the Postpartal Period and the Newborn Area

Frases para el Periodo Despues del Parto y el Area del Recien Nacido

Would you like to see your baby now?

¿Quiere ver a su bebé ahora?

Would you like me to help you feed your baby?

¿Quiere que le ayude a alimentarlo (la)?

Your baby needs a car seat to go home in.

El (la) bebé necesita un asiento para bebés en el automóvil.

Special Neonatal Needs

Necesidades del Recien Nacido

We are giving your baby oxygen.

Le vamos a dar oxígeno al (a la) bebé.

Your baby is having some problems breathing.

El (la) bebé tiene problemas al respirar.

Your baby needs extra help.

El (la) bebé necesita ayuda especial.

Your baby needs to go to a special care nursery.

El (la) bebé necesita ir a la sala de cuidados especiales para bebés.

Projected Recommendations for Isolation Precautions (CDC 1995)

The guidelines established by the Centers for Disease Control and Prevention (CDC) in 1995 have two levels of prevention—standard precautions, designed to be used with all clients, and transmission-based precautions, designed to be used with clients with suspected or confirmed infections with epidemiologically important organisms transmitted by airborne or droplet route or by direct contact with contaminated surfaces or dry skin. Section A of this Appendix (see page 352) describes the projected 1995 CDC guidelines, and section B (see page 355) summarizes the 1991 OSHA Bloodborne Pathogen Standard, which are an integral part of the Standard Precautions (CDC, 1995).

Section A   Projected Recommendations for Isolation Precautions (CDC 1995)

Type Precaution	Handwashing	Gloves	Gown	Mask, Eye Protection, Face Shield	Room Assignment of Client
Standard Precautions *To be used with all clients	Between all client contacts; immediately after removing gloves; after any contact with bodily fluids or secretions; or after any contact with contaminated items.	Nonsterile gloves worn when coming in contact with any bodily substances (saliva, urine, feces, blood, etc), mucous membranes, or nonintact skin.	Nonsterile, clean gown used during procedures in which splashing of bodily fluids is anticipated. Gown is discarded after tasks are finished.	Mask and eye protection or face shield worn whenever splashing or spraying of bodily fluids is probable.	Private room preferred if client is unable to maintain own hygiene or environmental control of room; otherwise room with multiple clients is acceptable.
Transmission-based precautions: Droplet *To be used for clients with known or suspected infections with microorganisms > 5 microns known to be	Same as above.	Same as above.	Same as above.	A mask is worn when working within three feet of the client.	Private room preferred if possible; if not possible a spatial separation of at least three feet must be maintained between client and other individuals such as other clients, visitors, etc.

transmitted by droplets from sneezing, talking, coughing, etc. **Transmission-based precautions: Airborne** *To be used for clients with known or suspected infection with microorganisms (≤ 5 microns) that can remain in the air or be dispersed widely by air currents.	Same as above.	Same as above.	Same as above.	A special mask (particulate respirator) is recommended for entering the rooms of clients with tuberculosis. Individuals who have never had varicella or rubeola should not enter the rooms of clients diagnosed with or suspected of having these infections.	Client room should have the following: • monitored negative air pressure • at least 6 air exchanges per hour • appropriate discharge of air from room. In addition, the door to room should be kept closed at all times. Client may be in a semi-private room with another client who has the same diagnosis. *Continued*

Section A continued

Type Precaution	Handwashing	Gloves	Gown	Mask, Eye Protection, Face Shield	Room Assignment of Client
Transmission-based precautions: Contact *To be used for clients with known or suspected infection with epidemiologically important microorganisms that can be transmitted by direct contact with the client or by indirect contact (for example, by touching objects or equipment in the client's room).	Same as above.	Use nonsterile, clean gloves in providing direct client care or during contact with potentially contaminated items.	Clean, nonsterile gown is recommended if contact with bodily substances, equipment, or surfaces is anticipated.	Same as for standard precautions.	Private room if possible.

Note: CDC Guidelines are extrapolated from: Draft guideline for isolation precautions in hospitals: notice of comment period. Federal Register 59(214):55552-55570. November 7, 1994. The final version of the guidelines may differ. Reviewed by Marguerite McMillan Jackson RN, Doctoral Candidate, CIC, FAAN. Administrative Director Medical Center Epidemiology Unit, University of California San Diego.

Section B Occupational Safety and Health Administration (OSHA) Bloodborne Pathogens Standard (1991)

The Bloodborne Pathogens Standard (1991) will be an integral part of the Standard Precautions (CDC 1995). This standard is to be used to prevent contact with blood or other materials that are potentially infectious. If the circumstance arises that body fluids are difficult to differentiate, all body fluids are considered potentially infectious. The essential elements of the Bloodborne Pathogens Standard are as follows:

- Handwashing guidelines should include:

  - Washing hands with soap and water prior to and immediately after contact with all clients and/or any contaminated items.
  - Hands are to be washed immediately after removing gloves.
  - Handwashing materials are to be made readily available in each work setting.

- Nonsterile, disposable gloves are to be worn whenever contact with blood or other potentially infectious body fluids may be anticipated. Gloves should be replaced if they are punctured or torn. Disposable gloves are to be used only once.

- Masks, eye protection, and face shields are to be worn whenever potentially contaminated material may be splashed, sprayed or spattered on the face, eyes, nose or mouth.

- Special care is to be taken when using or discarding sharp instruments (needles, scalpels or other sharp devices).

  - Needles are never to be recapped using two hands.
  - If the needle needs to be recapped, a one-handed 'scoop' technique may be used, or a special device for recapping may be used.
  - Used needles should not be removed from the syringe by hand.
  - Needles should not be manipulated, twisted or broken by hand.

- All sharps (needles, scalpels, and sharp disposable instruments) should be placed in an appropriate puncture-resistant container. The container should be clearly marked and/or color-coded, be leakproof on the sides and bottom, be located as close to the client as possible, be maintained in an upright position, and have a lid so spillage is not possible.

- During resuscitation, special disposable devices should be used as an alternative to the direct mouth-to-mouth method.

From: Department of Labor, Occupational Safety and Health Administration: Federal Register 56:64003-64182, Dec 6, 1991. Reviewed by Marguerite McMillan Jackson RN, Doctoral Candidate, CIC, FAAN. Administrative Director Medical Center, University of California San Diego.